I0028194

Routledge Revivals

Education for Childbirth and Parenthood

Originally published in 1980, the setting of this book is in the practicalities of teaching on labour wards, in antenatal clinics and in child health clinics. In such settings, health education about childbirth and parenthood is often an explicit, and always implicit, task for the health professional. The book results from several years' research on health service teaching methods and contains detailed studies of teaching in practice, in clinics, in classes and on wards, by midwives, health visitors, physiotherapists, doctors, National Childbirth Trust teachers and the writers of educational pamphlets. A number of transcripts of teaching sessions are presented to illustrate ways in which practitioners can develop more relevant and sensitive teaching strategies. The author shows that realistic goals are essential if the needs of learners, who are also problematically 'patients' and 'clients', are to be met.

The book offers insights into professional problems which voluntary organisations concerned with the health service and with educational work with parents, can use to help both themselves and their clients to make a more intelligent use of the facilities available. A more practical but critical philosophy of antenatal teaching is advocated, enabling all professionals involved to take a fresh look at their courses and clients.

Education for Childbirth and Parenthood

Elizabeth R. Perkins

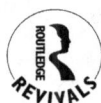

Routledge
Taylor & Francis Group

First published in 1980
by Croom Helm

This edition first published in 2018 by Routledge
2 Park Square, Milton Park, Abingdon, Oxon OX14 4RN

and by Routledge
711 Third Avenue, New York, NY 10017

Routledge is an imprint of the Taylor & Francis Group, an informa business

© 1980 Elizabeth R. Perkins

The right of Elizabeth R. Perkins to be identified as author of this work has been asserted by her in accordance with sections 77 and 78 of the Copyright, Designs and Patents Act 1988.

All rights reserved. No part of this book may be reprinted or reproduced or utilised in any form or by any electronic, mechanical, or other means, now known or hereafter invented, including photocopying and recording, or in any information storage or retrieval system, without permission in writing from the publishers.

Publisher's Note
The publisher has gone to great lengths to ensure the quality of this reprint but points out that some imperfections in the original copies may be apparent.

Disclaimer
The publisher has made every effort to trace copyright holders and welcomes correspondence from those they have been unable to contact.

A Library of Congress record exists under ISBN: 0709902735

ISBN: 978-0-8153-9884-4 (hbk)
ISBN: 978-1-351-17196-0 (ebk)
ISBN: 978-0-8153-9933-9 (pbk)

Education for Childbirth and Parenthood

ELIZABETH R. PERKINS

CROOM HELM LONDON

© 1980 Elizabeth R. Perkins
Croom Helm Ltd, 2-10 St John's Road, London SW11

British Library Cataloguing in Publication Data

Perkins, Elizabeth R
    Education for childbirth and parenthood.
    1. Childbirth — Study and teaching
    I. Title
    618.2'4   RG973

    ISBN 0-7099-0273-5

Typeset by Jayell Typesetting · London

CONTENTS

To all my adult students, who teach me how to teach

ACKNOWLEDGEMENTS

This book owes so much to the help of so many people that it is impossible to mention them all by name here. I would like to thank the many health service staff who have tolerated my presence in their clinics, classes and wards, have answered my questions, filled in my questionnaires, volunteered information and commented on my early drafts. In particular I owe a debt of gratitude to those who agreed to tape-record themselves, to discuss the results with me and to allow me to use extracts for publication. I would also like to thank those parents who have been prepared to suffer invasion of their privacy in the cause of research, and those parents and members of voluntary organisations who have helped me by commenting on my findings. If I still fail to understand the problems of professionals or patients, my errors are my own.

Research develops not only through data collection, but also through discussion; I would particularly like to thank Diana Stockwell, for her efforts with my midwifery education, and Ian McCafferty and my colleagues in the Leverhulme Health Education Project, for their share in many friendly arguments. During the period when the research for this book was undertaken, my co-authors and I were employed by the Leverhulme Health Education Project, Digby Anderson as Education Fellow and Nicholas Spencer as Medical Fellow. Digby Anderson and I thank Wesley Sharrock for permission to use the data on child health clinic interviews quoted in Chapter 7. We are all three grateful for the constant support and encouragement of the Director of the Leverhulme Health Education Project, Henry Fowler; for the remarkable patience and efficiency of Mary Pearson, Gillian Deave and Joy Caldwell in typing successive drafts of this book and the material on which it is based; and for the financial support of the Leverhulme Trust for our research.

Elizabeth Perkins
University of Nottingham

FOREWORD

I first met Elizabeth Perkins in 1976 when she wished to interview community midwives who had been involved in the care of some 40 recently delivered women who were the subject of health education research sponsored by the Leverhulme Trust.

As a result of that and other projects in this health district and others, I have developed a very happy working relationship with Elizabeth and a great respect for her work. She has brought a background of history and anthropology, and an ongoing experience in adult teaching to her research work, together with an obvious sympathy with and understanding of the problems confronting midwives and health visitors. She has always sought to work with us, so together we have learnt to question each other's assumptions, correct each other's misconceptions and develop each other's understanding of the need for learning and support of those for whom we care.

As a consequence, throughout the area, midwives and health visitors are using this work to reassess their objectives, change their teaching programmes and develop new skills in communication in order to improve their service to patients.

I hope that those involved in parentcraft teaching reading this book will, on recognising similar problems and experiences, gain similar insight into the issues involved and similar encouragement to search for solutions.

Diana Stockwell
Divisional Nursing Officer (Midwifery)
Central Notts Health District

1 PARENTS, PROSPECTIVE PARENTS AND HEALTH PROFESSIONALS

Teaching in Health Service Settings

This book is about teaching parents — and about patients learning. It is written for those health professionals, particularly in the maternity and child health services, who are concerned with teaching patients,[1] and for members of voluntary organisations and consumer groups who are interested in using or improving the opportunities available for parents to learn through contact with health service staff. It is not, however, either a manual of tips for health service teachers,[2] or a handbook for articulate consumers on how to beat the system.[3] Instead, this book consists of a series of studies of health service teaching in particular *settings*, in labour wards, antenatal classes and clinics, and by particular *methods*, through group work, through individual interviews, through in-patient care, and also indirectly, through leaflets. These settings, and these methods, have built-in strengths and weaknesses. Staff who teach, and parents who wish, as patients, to learn, could usefully take account of these strengths and weaknesses, so that they can together make the fullest use of the opportunities available in these settings, without making demands on them which are unrealistic.

The settings chosen for examination feature particular groups of practitioners: midwives, health visitors,[4] physiotherapists, doctors, and the writers of health educational literature. They also show members of a particular voluntary organisation, the National Childbirth Trust, both as providers and consumers of teaching. The NCT provides antenatal classes and educational literature to a small proportion of expectant parents, and in some parts of the country also provides advice on breast feeding and friendly postnatal support. These professional and voluntary groups have been chosen for study because they have a clearly stated and established interest in teaching as a part of their work; the possible exception here is the medical profession, and doctors' involvement in health education is discussed at length in Chapter 7.

The maternity and child health services have a long tradition of educational work, based on the demands of their patients' condition. Midwives, for example, require co-operation from pregnant women for the success of antenatal care. An informed woman in labour is likely to be an easier patient to care for, since fear and tension may distort the course of labour.[5] Physiotherapists, whether they are concerned with self-help techniques before the birth or with postnatal exercises afterwards, have no option but to teach, since clearly they cannot do exercises for patients. Similarly, midwives and health visitors cannot themselves look after babies for very long after birth, if at all, and therefore they teach mothers, and more recently fathers, to do so.

Teaching and Learning

The existence of well established health service teaching traditions justifies an examination of health service practice from an educational point of view. Education, however, involves activity on the part of the learner, as well as the teacher; indeed, the learner's activity is the more important, since it is possible for learning to take place without any direct teaching at all. Expectant and new parents, particularly women, are generally thought to be a particularly receptive group, willing or even eager to learn. The interest in teaching found among staff working with expectant or new parents in part reflects this willingness of their patients to learn. This very receptiveness may mislead health service teachers into concentrating on what they themselves wish to teach, rather than investigating what parents wish to learn, and what preconceptions, existing knowledge, or misinformation they bring with them to the encounter with professional staff. Good teaching is not achieved by treating learners as a passive audience; it does involve expecting and encouraging learners to take an active part in their own learning. Establishing links between old knowledge and new, or between established behaviour and possible new patterns, is part of the learning process. Teachers can make this easier for learners; but to do so they need to know something about individual learners' existing ideas and behaviour. This is easier in some situations than others, and with some patients than with others; the implications of encouraging active learning in practice is a recurrent theme of the following chapters.

Encouragement may be of particular importance to patients who are not very articulate, or lack self-confidence. Studies which document patient dissatisfaction with communication in the health service[6] frequently include sketches of that apparently puzzling phenomenon, the patient who wants information but does not like to bother the staff by asking for it. One reason for this reluctance may be that in practice, in the health service, the initiative mostly rests with the professionals. They know the usual procedures. They can provide, or deny, the opportunity to ask questions without obviously disrupting the smooth flow of a clinic, or an antenatal class. They can assess more readily than inexperienced patients what is practical in a particular setting at a particular time, and because patients know this, they may well expect the opportunities for questions to be made by the professionals. Health service staff should be aware of the power they wield, so that they may use it in the interests of the individual patients they serve, and also so that where possible they can hand back responsibility for learning to the patients from whom it came. For learning is finally something which patients must do for themselves, and a passive trust in the benevolence and wisdom of professional staff, however justified this may be,[7] will not foster active learning.

The Advantages of 'Awkward' Patients

Passive patients encourage professionals to retain responsibility, and thus to discourage active learning. Since it may be easier to deal with patients who do not ask awkward questions, and who do as they are told, at least when the staff are present, professionals may not always find it convenient to encourage patient initiative. It is here that articulate, possibly 'awkward' patients, pressure groups and voluntary organisations, have a value in encouraging good teaching practice within the health service. They may infuriate practitioners, but they do provide a continuous reminder that there are other things for a patient to resemble than a door mat. Staff who learn ways of meeting the needs of the articulate may also find that they can use what they have learned to encourage more passive patients, or to remove barriers to patient initiative of which they were not previously aware, because no one had challenged these barriers before. Professionals can do much to improve patient education in the health service on their own. They can do more where patients help them to change their approach to learning and teaching. Learners have to make some effort to work with teachers, particularly where teachers have other things on their minds besides teaching, like the demands of clinical practice.

The Role of Patient Organisations

Voluntary groups can do more than act as hairshirts for professionals. In some instances they may provide an alternative education service, as

does the National Childbirth Trust. Some health service staff who are
critical of the NCT are inclined to see it as a threat to their own educational provision; they point out, with some justification, that it caters
for the middle classes, and criticise its teaching on the basis of the,
possibly 'awkward', patients they meet who have attended NCT classes.
'Awkward' patients, as we have seen, have their uses, and material relevant to an assessment of NCT teaching is included in Chapters 2 and 3.
Any voluntary organisation which provides classes for a clientele with
special needs, whether it caters for intellectual career women in their
thirties, unmarried mothers, or, in our multi-racial society, Mirpuri-
speakers, may be a help to the health service staff by coping with the
unusual type of patient who is difficult to deal with in the usual antenatal class. If the NCT provides well for one of these special groups, this
justifies its existence. Voluntary organisations need not attempt to
cater for all patients; that is the role of the health service.

Further, voluntary organisations catering for special groups may act
as pioneers. They have great freedom to experiment; they have, almost
by definition, enthusiastic staff, whether paid or unpaid, and a committed membership. They have an understanding of the patients' points of
view which it may take considerable effort for a professional to acquire.
They can therefore try new ways of meeting the needs of their own
members which may later be of use to health service staff. Borrowing
methods from enthusiastic self-help groups however, must involve some
caution. They may suit the membership of that group, but they will not
necessarily suit everyone. Local face-to-face groups may take on a particular social character which excludes others.[8] This may or may not be
because the members are 'middle class', whatever that over-worked
term means in a particular context. Professionals considering trying out
new ideas used by voluntary groups will obviously bear in mind the
context in which they are then being used, and that to which they are
to be transferred.

Voluntary groups can help professionals to a better understanding of
patients' needs, and can contribute some alternative methods of
meeting them. Equally, voluntary organisations can learn from, and
about, professionals. The more understanding they have of the nature
of professional traditions, and the particular characteristics of professional working settings, the more capable they will be of helping their
members to use the learning opportunities in the health service to the
best advantage, without causing unnecessary friction. Professionals may
be able to work with voluntary organisations towards improvements
which both groups would wish to see. If this fruitful co-operation is to

materialise, however, an understanding of one another's strengths and limitations is highly desirable, if not essential.

The Uses of Local Studies

This book is based on a series of local studies, limited in both area and scale. The nature and uses of this type of evidence deserve some preliminary consideration, for local studies may contribute to two different types of examination of professional practice. In the locality where the work is undertaken, such studies may provide local health workers with material to assess their practice in terms of their own priorities, and, where necessary to act accordingly. The research on which this book is based has been discussed with managers and field staff and has contributed to that self-examination which is a part of truly professional work.[9] In addition, the insights and experience of local professional staff have been of great value in the analysis of the material.

The alternative use of local studies is a more general one, and is the rationale for this book. There is no intention to imply that the results of these studies would be repeated in every ward, clinic or antenatal class up and down the country. Detailed, small scale studies instead enable the research worker to look for the dynamics of the situation, for the pressures operating on individual staff which lead them to behave in the way they do.[10] Some of these pressures are undoubtedly local or individual: particular personalities, liaison problems, shortage of money, or design of buildings. But to try to explain good practice, or to explain away bad practice on these grounds does less than justice to other staff who manage well in difficult conditions. Explanations based on these individual or local characteristics are only partial. If, for example, staff are tired, or very rushed, they are obviously more likely to make mistakes. But the sort of mistakes they make will be determined not only by their individual personalities, but also by the ordering of professional priorities which they have learned and which may have become instinctive. The doctor who consults the midwife, but fails to speak to the woman in labour when he is called in at the end of a long period of duty, may behave like this because he is tired. But his bad manners also reflect a belief that talking to the patient is an optional extra. For him, the really important part of the job is to find out why the midwife thinks his presence is needed, and to do something about it. It is not enough to say that the man is tired, or to say

that he is rude. Both may be true, in this situation. Neither is an
adequate explanation of his behaviour. An understanding of his professional priorities is necessary for a more nearly complete picture.

Similarly, small scale studies make it possible to look closely at the
problems of patients in particular settings, and in particular that of the
patient who does not like to bother the staff. Staff who are only too
willing to give information on request may find research which demon-
strates patient dissatisfaction with this aspect of health service care
both hard to accept and hard to act on if accepted. They are already
willing to teach, and it is not easy to distinguish a patient who is too
shy to ask questions from a patient who has no questions. Small scale
studies may reveal barriers to patient initiative which could be dismant-
led, or circumvented, once staff are aware that they exist. For example,
a patient's belief that staff are too busy to teach may be true; it may
also be based on a misunderstanding of how demanding the staff's
activity is. Some jobs require concentration, but experienced staff can
quite easily chat to patients as they put out or clear away equipment,
or undertake routine examinations. The inexperienced patient may not
realise this, and thus see no opening to ask a question, or raise a problem. Teaching in the health service, in a way that responds to individuals' needs, has something to do with having a caring and responsive
personality, but it may have a lot more to do with making apparent
that willingness to care, to teach and to respond to individual need, to
particular people, in particular settings, in particular ways. There are
technical skills involved as well as personal characteristics; small scale
studies can help to identify what those technical skills may be, so that
they can be taught and practised more effectively in the future.

For teaching in health service settings has distinctive features, related
to the blending of teaching with medical or nursing care. Staff have
access to individual clinical information on patients, and can use this to
relate each patient's condition to that of the average patient. This
information can be used in assessing the needs of each individual and
attempting to meet them. For this reason no final substitute for
teaching by health service staff is to be found in work by school
teachers, by voluntary organisations, or through leaflets. Such work
may be valuable, but it cannot take into account the circumstances of
this patient at this time with this particular clinical condition. This
information is only available when health service staff and patients
meet; it is through the pooling of their joint store of information that
the needs of an individual patient can be established, and the staff and
patient together can make efforts to see that appropriate care and

appropriate learning take place. This process is not simple, either to understand or to carry out, and it is in the belief that an improved understanding of the process can lead to improved practice that this book is written.

Notes

1. For a discussion of the implications of patient status for the learning process, see Chapter 8.

2. Books which could be used in this way are already available; see, for example, M. Williams and D. Booth, *Antenatal Education: Guidelines for Teachers* (Churchill Livingstone, Edinburgh, 1974); Sheila Kitzinger, *Education and Counselling for Childbirth* (Baillière Tindall, London, 1977); Patricia Hassid, *Textbook for Childbirth Educators* (Harper & Row, Hagerstown, Maryland, 1978).

3. Books which approximate to this stance include: Christine Beels, *The Childbirth Book* (Turnstone Books, London, 1978); Jane and John Lennane, *Hard Labour* (Gollancz, London, 1974); Sheila Kitzinger, *The Good Birth Guide* (Fontana, Glasgow, 1979).

4. Health visitors are trained nurses, with some obstetric nursing experience and a year's training for work in the community. Many, though not all, qualified as midwives before they trained as health visitors. They undertake no practical nursing, and instead have responsibility for educational and advisory work. In the past their work was concerned with mothers and young children, but in recent years their responsibilities have broadened; most health visitors still spend much time in work with young families, but schemes of attachment to specific general practitioners have encouraged more work with other sections of the population.

5. The classic formulation of this theory is contained in Grantly Dick Read, *Natural Childbirth* (Heinemann, London, 1933).

6. Reviews of literature on communication between health professionals and patients may be found in Debra L. Roter, 'Patient Participation in the Patient-provider Interaction: The Effects of Patient Question Asking on the Quality of Interaction, Satisfaction and Compliance', *Health Education Monographs* (Winter 1977), p. 281; and J.M. Clark and Lisbeth Hockey, *Research for Nursing: A Guide for the Enquiring Nurse* (HM & M, Aylesbury, 1979), pp. 78-92.

7. Isabel E.R. Menzies, 'The Functioning of Social Systems and a Defence against Anxiety', Tavistock Pamphlet no. 3 (Tavistock Institute, of Human Relations, London, 1970), comments on the way in which patients may encourage staff to take over all responsibility for them.

8. For a critical look at self-help groups, see Stuart Henry, 'The Dangers of Self-help Groups', *New Society* (22 June 1978) p. 654.

9. See the Foreword to this book.

10. For a discussion of the importance of small scale studies, see Margaret Stacey with Hilary Homans, 'The Sociology of Health and Illness; Its Present State, Future Prospects and Potential for Health Research', *Sociology*, vol. 12 (1978), p. 281.

2 THE LABOUR WARD AS AN EDUCATIONAL SETTING

The Theoretical Case for Education

A woman who gives birth in hospital is faced with several different types of unfamiliarity. If it is her first pregnancy the sensations of labour will be unknown; even in second or subsequent pregnancies, the pattern of labour may be unfamiliar, varying from earlier experiences because of the position of the baby, the presence or absence of obstetric complications, or the type of management employed by the staff. Equipment involved in the management of labour, or standing in the corner of the room in case of need, is likely to be unfamiliar. It is unlikely that a woman will have previously met the staff responsible for her care, and several different members of staff will probably be involved, because of meal breaks and shift changes. She is also likely to be unfamiliar with the working patterns of hospital, so that the comings and goings of staff may make no sense without specific explanations. Finally, she may never have seen the labour ward before.

All this unfamiliarity at first suggests that there is a great need for teaching on the labour ward, so that women can be helped to understand their situation, and not to fear the unknown. Since fear is believed to disrupt normal labour,[1] midwives have a practical as well as a humanitarian reason for wishing to dispel it. In addition, there is a case for teaching women techniques which they can use to cope with their sensations. Finally, it can be argued that women have a right to explanations; they have a responsibility for the baby's welfare which transcends that of hospital staff, and therefore a right, or a duty, to be involved in decisions made about labour and delivery. This argument has been advanced with considerable force by Haire, writing from an American background:

> To withhold information as to the possible complications of obstetrical medication is to delude the mother into assuming that there are no risks involved.
> We must bear in mind that it is the mother who must ultimately bear the major emotional burden of a damaged or impaired child, even if that child is institutionalised. Under normal conditions no one should usurp the mother's prerogative by placing her unborn or

newborn infant at a possible disadvantage without her informed consent.[2]

These essentially theoretical arguments, however, sound much less convincing when they are set against the realities of life on the labour ward. Teaching requires time, and this may not be available. This may be particularly true of teaching self-help techniques. Even giving information, either to dispel fear, or to make informed decision-making possible, may be made more difficult by the demands of practical midwifery. Since work-load is unpredictable, except for inductions, and deliveries require immediate action, teaching patients in early labour may have to be abandoned in favour of more immediately urgent tasks. There are, therefore, practical difficulties inherent in the working situation of the staff, not all of which can be dispelled by exhortations to do more teaching, or even by in-service training programmes to teach them how to teach more effectively.

It has been argued in Chapter 1 that education should involve activity on the part of the learner, and here too there are considerable difficulties. There are midwives who argue that self-help techniques can be taught on the labour ward,[3] but others would say that patients in labour are in no fit state to learn. A woman in pain, probably short of sleep, and in an unfamiliar and possibly frightening setting, is unlikely to be an alert and active learner, even if she would benefit from the skills or the knowledge which someone is trying to teach her. Clearly there are problems for the learner, as well as for the teacher.

Possible Responses

There are two main possible approaches to the problem posed by the theoretical case for education on the labour ward, and the manifest problems in practice. One is to argue that two types of action could be taken before the woman arrives. First, self-help techniques could be taught in antenatal classes, where hospital work patterns could also be explained. The unfamiliarity of the labour ward and the machinery it contains could be in part dispelled by organising guided tours round the ward. Secondly, where circumstances permit, the rooms could be made as homelike as possible, and thus more familiar, with equipment out of sight until it is needed, and soft furnishings at least in the first stage rooms. This sort of solution is only partial. The first one depends on all the women attending antenatal classes where teaching is of a high standard, both in method and in content. Attendance at classes appears from the few specific studies available to average about 45 per cent[4] of pregnant women. Studies of antenatal classes included in this volume suggest that standards of teaching may vary widely, and that problems may arise in adapting some physical preparation techniques to the reality of labour. While previous attendance at classes provides a woman and the staff who care for her with a foundation on which they can build, it thus seems unlikely that it will solve all their problems; where women have not attended classes, an alternative approach is needed anyway. Since at least some women who do not attend classes regret their inability to do so and provide convincing reasons for it,[5] this approach cannot legitimately be one of blaming the victim. Further, even where women attend classes which provide soundly based and well taught preparation for *childbirth*, they may not receive much preparation for *hospital*, if the staff concerned are not themselves familiar with details or procedures. Finally, for many hospitals it will not be possible, either for financial reasons, or because of the demands of medical technology, to tackle the problem from the other end, and adapt the hospital to resemble a home.

A second approach to the theoretical case for education is to admit the problem of multiple unfamiliarity, but to argue that an educational solution is inappropriate, particularly for women who have received no previous organised education about childbirth. Instead, pain can be eased by drugs and reassurance, and unfamiliarity with the staff, hospital setting and routine by the provision of warm supportive care from the staff, and/or the presence of a person well known to the labouring woman, usually her husband. Decision-making, in this view, is an unfair demand to make on a woman in labour. She will, of course, be asked for her consent to various procedures, but requests will be phrased in such a way as to make it clear that she is not really expected to think; instead, she can safely trust the judgement of the staff. This approach, like the earlier one, may also have limitations if applied to all women all the time. Here the categories of women from whom it may be inappropriate are less clearly defined, but that such women exist can be demonstrated from the complaints about lack of information, removal of choice, and the provision of ineffective reassurance instead. Such comments come from women's groups, voluntary organisations concerned with the maternity services, and also from some research studies.[6]

Both these approaches can be justified as partial solutions to the theoretical case for education on the labour ward and the practical difficulties in responding to this case. They even appear to dovetail; it would be tempting to divide women into two groups, those who go to classes, and can therefore be treated as suitable cases for teaching, building on previous work, and those women who do not attend classes, who really want reassurance and support in labour. Once this is explicitly stated, however, it sounds less appealing; midwives are well aware that women in labour react very differently, and that in addition their needs will change as labour progresses.[7] Rigid categories are clearly inappropriate for such an individual process.

Wants and Needs — The Problem of Assessment

The assessment of individual needs is a complicated process. No one except the woman herself can know what she feels that she needs. This lack of direct access to felt needs is a problem for midwives and for research workers. Asking women about the sort of care they would like in labour is bedevilled by the problem of expectations; women who expect the bare minimum of physical care are unlikely to demand much more than this at the time, and may express complaints after-wards with some hesitancy, even to outside research workers.[8] This problem has also been found in studies of doctor-patient interviews;[9] patients greatly appreciated explanations, but did not expect them. A guide to standards of care which come closest to meeting patients' needs could usefully be based on patients' praise for care they received, rather than a theoretical outline from them of the care they would like.

Donna Shields,[10] studying care in labour in the United States in relation to patient satisfaction, isolated supportive care as being the form of care found most helpful in labour. The main components within this category were: the presence of the nurse; explanation or teaching; and reassurance, comfort or concern. Explanations or teaching, she concluded, were partly a matter of telling the patient how she was progressing, and what the staff were doing, but also included teaching techniques for pushing or breathing during contractions. She concluded that this was not merely a matter of reassuring the patient that all was going well, but also included an element not isolated in previous research, defined by her as 'guidance or coaching in labour'. While this work is based on an analysis of nursing, rather than mid-wifery care, it clearly has implications for midwifery practice. If some form of teaching is a major component of good supportive care, and this is much appreciated by patients, adequate solutions to the theoreti-cal case for education must incorporate some teaching by labour ward staff, as well as using the alternatives of preparation beforehand and the reassuring presence of a midwife during labour.

Those who are present with a woman in labour have a different sort of access to information about need from that obtained in research. While it is individual, it is not direct information; it is filtered through the patient's efforts to arrange for her needs to be met. This is information on *expressed* needs. A midwife in charge of a case has, in addition, her own professional judgement about the woman's clinical condition, establishing *normative* need.[11] This professional assessment may or may not coincide with the woman's views of her needs. A further complicating factor in a midwife's assessment of a woman's wants, or her needs, according to clinical criteria, is that she has responsibilities which may interfere with this assessment; these responsibilities may be to other patients, or to the smooth running of the institution in which she works. Some wants, of some women, may be seen by a midwife to be a distraction from her other patients, or contrary to ward routine, hospital policy or consultants' preferences. Inconvenient wants, expressed weakly by patients, may not be perceived at all. A midwife's assessment of her patients' needs thus passes through two filters: that of her professional judgement, and that of the patient's efforts to express it. The position of an observer on the ward is rather easier; such a person has no clinical responsibility, and no other patients, and can attend only to the problem of the expression of needs. Material from an observation study of social interaction on the labour ward[12] is therefore useful in considering the place of teaching on the labour ward in relation to other forms of supportive care.

The Source of the Evidence

The data presented in this chapter represent a small proportion of the evidence collected during a study undertaken in two maternity units, involving observation of women in labour and staff at work.[13]

The observer's presence on the labour ward was clearly an anomaly for both patients and staff. She always asked the patient's permission to stay with her in labour, and made it clear that she would go, temporarily or permanently, if requested to do so. She wore a hospital gown over street clothes, as husbands did, after realising that the theatre dress she wore on her first visits contradicted for patients her repeated statements that she was not a midwife. Her efforts to clarify the situation for patients did not preserve her from twice being mistaken for a doctor by the staff! The observer carried a shorthand notebook and wrote notes as events developed. She found some difficulty in

developing a short explanation of her presence which was comprehensible to both patients and staff, and at the same time bore some relationship to her purposes. She finally settled on a description of her
interest in preparation for childbirth and parenthood, the problem of
preparing people for hospital life, and her ignorance of hospital patterns
of work — thus her need to 'come and see what happened'. This usually
satisfied patients, who went on to ask her about her own childbearing
plans and the effect on her of watching women in labour. Staff were,
understandably, more preoccupied with what she was writing in her
notebook!

The Maternity Units Involved

Both units were modern, set in the grounds of a larger hospital, but had
different physical structures and served different types of communities.
Unit A served a population drawn from small industrial towns and the
rural communities around, while Unit B catered also for university
women, inner city 'problem families' and immigrant communities with
language difficulties. Unit A had been built with separate first stage and
delivery rooms, whereas women admitted to Unit B remained in the
same bed, in the same room, throughout their labour.

The first stage rooms in Unit A, and the rooms in Unit B, were provided with patterned curtains and toning paint on the walls, an easy
chair for husbands and a bedside table for odds and ends; this was
partly occupied by hospital odds and ends, like electric fans to reduce
the temperature in Unit B, and carafes and glasses of water. The
woman's belongings were kept in a trolley in Unit A (the top of which
formed the bedside table) and in a basket in Unit B. In Unit A the
woman wore her own nightdress; in Unit B she changed into a hospital
gown on admission, but this was coloured and flowered, and the husband of one of the study women mistakenly admired her 'new nightdress'! The hospitals had thus made some effort in the direction of
reducing unfamiliarity by attention to the trappings of the labour ward,
but it would be impossible to describe either place as homelike. In Unit
B the equipment for emergencies or for delivery was extremely obvious
and there seemed to be a lot of it. In Unit A this equipment was kept in
the delivery room, and therefore out of sight for most of the time, but
the alternative view was a bare wall, or a clock — and the clocks were,
according to the staff, always wrong or stopped. In addition, most of
Unit A's rooms were not in any way soundproofed, and the staff in
both units frequently left doors open, adding to the impression of lack
of privacy.

Both units had made considerable efforts to tackle the problem of unfamiliarity by preparing the women, rather than the building. Each provided relaxation classes for a small proportion of the women admitted, and many of their patients attended classes held in the community. Unit A arranged visits to the labour ward for community classes, usually with an accompanying community midwife or health visitor, and also had a policy of arranging tours for individuals on request. Unit B accepted visits from community classes, but also held open evenings where women, or couples, could come without appointment, see a film and be shown round the unit.

When women arrived in labour, the hospital admission patterns varied. Unit A usually arranged for one of the staff who would subsequently care for the woman to admit her; Unit B treated this duty as a specialist one, to be carried out by the sister in charge, assisted by nursing auxiliaries. Both used admission rooms separate from the labour ward itself; Unit B's admission suite had apparently become a thoroughfare for staff, and on occasion staff would walk through the bathroom when it was in use. Both units had similar procedures to undertake, including taking a history, checking blood pressure, listening to the foetal heart, carrying out an internal examination, timing contractions, preparing a label to go on the woman's wrist, shave (full shave in Unit A, half shave in Unit B), enema and bath. After the admission routine was completed, providing the woman was believed to be in established labour, she was escorted to her labour room and settled in. At this point, in Unit B, she would meet the member(s) of staff who would be responsible for her care, and if her husband had brought her in he would be recalled from the husbands' waiting room to rejoin his wife. Both hospitals had a policy of encouraging husbands to be present in labour and at delivery.

Where labour was to be induced the women were normally admitted to the antenatal ward the day before, brought down to the labour ward in the morning and, in Unit B, ushered straight to their rooms to meet their midwives. In Unit A they were more likely to wait in the waiting room, with a member of staff where possible, until the doctors arrived; inductions had to be carried out in delivery rooms, since first stage rooms were not equipped for the procedure, and thus they could not be settled in 'their' first stage rooms until afterwards. They would, however, first meet 'their' midwife who would help with the induction procedure. Husbands were not present during inductions. Both units had set up systems which were intended to tackle the issue of unfamiliarity of patients with staff through a policy of patient allocation on the labour ward; thus each patient would have at least one particular person assigned to care for her, until change of shift. In practice there were often two people, a sister and a comparatively inexperienced staff midwife, or pupil midwife; sometimes a medical student was also allocated to a patient, especially in Unit B. Both units in addition had overlapping shifts in the afternoon, so that there could be four people involved with one patient at once, particularly at Unit B where there were more full-time staff. Clinical responsibility was, of course, clearly assigned. Unit A was less well staffed; Unit B, on the other hand, had the possibility of far more confusion for the patient precisely because there were more staff.

Case Studies

From the mass of material collected, two case studies have been chosen to illustrate the problems and possibilities of teaching on labour wards, in units where considerable thought had already been applied to reducing unfamiliarity by advance preparation, both of the women and the wards. These particular case studies have not been selected on the grounds that they are typical either of women in labour or of their care in these particular units; indeed, it should be obvious from the account of the observer's experience and background that such a judgement would be out of place. Instead, these two examples have been chosen to illustrate the limitations of the two partial solutions to the case for education outlined earlier, those of preparation beforehand, and supportive care during labour.

Mrs X was a woman of 30 expecting her first baby. Her husband was an executive who arrived at the hospital with a case of papers and demonstrated, at least to the staff, his intention of doing some work during the early stages of labour. In fact he never touched the work he had brought. They had tried to arrange to go to classes at the hospital, found there had been a muddle over booking so that Mrs X could expect to have the baby before the end of the course, and had therefore travelled some distance, in bad weather, to attend National Childbirth Trust classes as well, though they were unable to make arrangements in time to complete this course either. The NCT classes were open to both parents, and Mr X did attend with his wife. They completed four weeks of each course before Mrs X went into labour and was admitted to Unit A, with her husband in attendance from the beginning. Mrs X clearly corresponds to the first partial solution. She and her husband had taken some trouble to arrange preparation for childbirth classes. They had not visited the maternity unit, since they had been expecting to be able to go with the hospital class during the next week. Since any blame for their inadequate preparation for hospital would appear to lie with the health service rather than with Mr and Mrs X, this couple provide an illustration of the unwisdom of dismissing unprepared patients as being uninterested in education. While their preparation was incomplete, they had a foundation of knowledge on which further teaching could, theoretically, be built.

Mrs Y was also 30, but was expecting her third child. Her earlier children were aged nine and six, and she had then had a series of miscarriages. Her husband, a postman, came in to see her when his work was over for the day, hoping he would be able to stay for the birth; he had been unable to stay with her for the birth of either of the other children. She had been admitted to the antenatal ward of Unit B two days before, and said that she had had no sleep the first night and only four hours sleep the second night, despite being given sleeping tablets. She said that the extra day in hospital had been arranged because she agreed to be available for the final examinations of medical students, before her induction for post-maturity on the following day. She had not attended classes either in this pregnancy or the two previous full-term ones, saying that she was 'not bothered' about labour, and that induction was the worst thing (her second baby was also induced). She told the observer that she was deaf in one ear. Mrs Y thus might not appear to be a promising case for teaching, since she had made no effort to prepare herself for childbirth beforehand, relying instead on her previous childbearing experience.

There are, of course, other ways in which Mrs X and Mrs Y may be contrasted. They differed in social class, in childbearing experience, in their husbands' ability to be present throughout the labour, and in the way in which their labours began. It can be argued that the last distinction, between induced and non-induced births, may in practice be less important than it is in theory. When women who have started labour spontaneously are admitted to hospital they may well be expected to co-operate with management techniques which include the artificial rupture of membranes, the acceleration of labour by means of a syntocinon drip, and external or internal monitoring of the foetus. The practical effects may thus be identical to an induced labour. Class, childbearing experience, husband's presence, and induction do, however, represent other variables which staff could use to distinguish between patients and which the reader could adopt now. The case for a perspective based on the patients' interest in education for childbirth is that, unlike the other variables, it is not a fixed entity; during labour this interest may increase or decrease, and it is a factor which staff may themselves affect. It is one of practical relevance to staff in their management of patients, amenable to their influence if not to their control. While it is by no means the only perspective available to staff or researchers, it is grounded both in the professional traditions of midwives and in the options open to childbearing women. It is therefore a perspective worth investigating.

The Course of Labour: Unfamiliarity in Practice

Mrs X arrived at Unit A at approximately 1.05 p.m., and the observer joined her in the admission room half an hour later. At this stage she was losing fluid; the staff midwife admitting her said that her cervix was six centimetres dilated and her forewaters intact. The staff midwife had earlier told her that she would probably need a drip to speed matters on, and expressed surprise and pleasure that Mrs X's labour was progressing so well. Her forewaters were ruptured, and an external monitor was used to monitor the baby's heartbeat. At 6.00 p.m. Mrs X began to experiment with Entonox (gas and oxygen); at 6.30 p.m. a vaginal examination showed her cervix to be eight centimetres dilated. At 8.30 p.m. the Entonox was exchanged for another inhalant analgesic, Penthrane. At the next vaginal examination, between 10.30 and 11.00 p.m., her cervix was fully dilated (ten centimetres), and her son was born just before midnight. Her husband (and the observer) were present throughout labour, apart from breaks for meals, drinks, telephone calls and, for the husband, admission routines and internal examinations.

The observer first joined Mrs Y in Unit B as her induction was about to start, at 9.05 a.m.; Mrs Y had been down on the labour ward for about half an hour before this. During the course of the doctor's examination the baby's head became free of the pelvis; instead of the planned artificial rupture of membranes followed by the use of a syntocinon drip, Mrs Y spent the morning with a drip only, waiting for the baby's head to re-enter the pelvis. At 3.30 p.m. she was examined by the registrar, her cervix was found to be four centimetres dilated, and her membranes were ruptured. A clip was attached to the baby's head for later use, and two external monitoring devices applied to check on the baby's heartbeat and the mother's contractions. The

contraction monitor did not record well and was removed; problems
with monitoring devices persisted throughout the labour, with different machines being wheeled in and out. At 4.35 p.m. Mrs Y had an
injection of pethidine; at 5.25 p.m. an extra glucose drip was put up
for her. At 5.30 p.m. she was examined internally, and the syntocinon
drip was discontinued because her complaints of persistent pain led the
staff to fear the risk of a ruptured uterus. At 7.30 p.m. a further
vaginal examination showed that Mrs Y had a swollen cervix because
she had been pushing before it was fully dilated. Sister therefore
suggested epidural analgesia, and at 8.15 p.m. the procedure was
started. Unfortunately the first attempt was a failure, and a second was
underway at 8.50 p.m., when the observer left. Mr Y arrived at 3.00 p.m.,
left at 5.35 p.m. and returned at 7.40 p.m., having decided not to use
the hospital canteen for a meal but to go into town instead. He left the
room during internal examinations and during the epidural procedures.
The baby arrived soon after the observer left, with no complications.

The facts given above should be taken as a series of fixed points for
reference, rather than as an attempt at exhaustive clinical summary.
These facts will now be related to the theoretical case for education
made at the beginning of this chapter. Mrs X, expecting her first baby,
had therefore no practical familiarity with the sensations of labour,
despite her efforts to learn the theory from NHS and NCT classes. She
had not had a trip round the labour ward, and had therefore not seen
the equipment or the sort of room she would occupy. She experienced
a shift change, at 9.00 p.m., and before 9.00 p.m. the staff midwife allocated to care for her had an extended period of absence from the
labour ward while she showed a party round another part of the
maternity unit. Mrs Y was used to labour, and, indeed, was induced at
the end of her previous pregnancy, though this was by artificial rupture
of membranes alone, and a syntocinon drip was therefore unfamiliar.
She said, however, that the course of this labour was different from
that of her previous labours, and this difference caused her considerable
distress. She had previously given birth in hospital, but not in this particular unit, which was new since her last full-term pregnancy. She too
experienced the effects of shift change, having a change at 1.00 p.m.,
when new staff took over responsibility although the previous staff
were still on the ward, and another at 9.00 p.m. when she was in very
late first stage labour. In many ways, therefore, Mrs X and Mrs Y could
be seen as having similar problems with unfamiliarity, increasingly
similar as Mrs Y's labour progressed and her sensations became more
and more different from those she recalled from her previous

experience. It does not, however, follow that because Mrs X and Mrs Y had similar problems, they wanted similar solutions — or that they set about finding these solutions in similar ways.

The Search for Solutions

The evidence on which midwife or observer can base an assessment of what a woman wants is the same as evidence about how she tries to get it. Both depend on a judgement about what is, or is not, an expression of need; the research worker merely has more opportunities to observe possible expressions of need. The simplest evidence is, of course, a direct question or request for information or help. The other extreme lies in non-verbal communication, oblique expressions of need which are difficult to identify with certainty. The woman who stares at her husband's empty chair, or at the Entonox mask as it is removed from her may be expressing a wish for the return of the person or object concerned, the familiar gesture of rubbing the place where the pain is may be an expression of a wish that someone else would rub it instead, particularly when, as with backache, it is rather difficult to manage this oneself. Such oblique expressions of need — if such they are — create problems of uncertainty both for midwife and research worker. Here, however, the midwife has an advantage. If she is not sure whether an action, or a look, is an expression of need, she can find out by asking, or by offering the help she thinks may be wanted. The research worker should not do this; she is in no position to offer help, except of the most basic kind, like passing glasses of water, and if she does offer help, she is increasing her impact on the situation and affecting the likelihood of the woman doing something else about her problem. Inhibiting helpful impulses entirely was found to be impossible, but the observer did try to reduce them to a minimum, and did not use offering help as a method of finding out what women wanted. She was therefore limited to her observations of direct expressions of need, and of others' efforts to convert indirect expressions into direct ones by asking questions or offering help, and to interpretations of communications, verbal and non-verbal, which were sometimes difficult to interpret with clarity without the ability to offer help. This sort of evidence is the basis of this account of Mrs X and Mrs Y, their difficulties in labour, and their search for appropriate solutions.

Information

Both Mrs X and Mrs Y saw some of their problems with unfamiliarity as soluble through a quest for information. Both had a period at the beginning of the observation where their requests to the staff were dominated by this quest. In Mrs X's case this was particularly marked; over the first hour and a half, when she was already six centimetres dilated, she asked a string of questions relating to admission procedure, the effects of the rupture of membranes, staff routine, hospital layout and monitors, and if necessary persisted until she was satisfied that she understood. For example, during admission she was told by the midwife that a solution would be used to wash her before her pubic hair was shaved; she asked 'What solution's that?', and was given the technical name. To this she replied, in an amused tone of voice, 'I'm none the wiser now' and was given an alternative answer 'a sterile solution', which seemed to satisfy her. She did not confine herself to the direct question and, here, the oblique follow-up, but took active steps to satisfy her wish for information. When she was taken to the first stage room to be settled in, she asked where the delivery room was, explaining that she had not been on a tour of the labour suite. The midwife told her that it was next door, pointing to the connecting door, and Mrs X got off the bed to go and have a look, saying that she had thought it would be a long way away, quite separate from the first stage rooms. The staff midwife allocated to care for her until shift change adapted successfully to Mrs X's persistent search for detailed information, which far outweighed her one request for extra pillows so that she could sit up easily, her two requests related to her husband's presence and need to wear a gown, and her request for confirmation that he could take photographs after the baby was born. The effects of this adaptation could be seen later in labour; at about 4.30 p.m. Mrs X said that she felt sick, and the midwife offered her a white liquid, saying 'Drink this, it is magnesium trisilicate'. As Mrs X hesitated, the midwife followed this by telling her that it would neutralise the acid in the stomach. The midwife interpreted her hesitation as an oblique expression of a need for information, and supplied the information in response to this. Mrs X drank the magnesium trisilicate, and the midwife told her that feeling sick was 'a good sign, a sign of progress'. This last comment from the midwife is a good example of the way in which the provision of information may merge into the provision of reassurance. We shall return to this point later.

Mrs Y also expressed a need for information. She was, however, somewhat ineffective in doing so. She experienced an unsuccessful attempt to break her membranes, which caused the doctor responsible some concern. The doctor had accompanied her actions with a running commentary, 'The baby's head keeps floating away from me, that's why I'm having trouble . . . the head's disappeared altogether' (at this point Mrs Y said 'Oh'). 'He's become disengaged, that's all . . . I think he's saying I've got fed up . . . let's see if he's come back . . . No . . . I'll have to see Mr — [registrar] . . . does it feel engaged from the top end?' (to sister). At this point the doctor left the room in search of the registrar, and as she left Mrs Y asked a question ending in 'up'. The tone of voice was interrogative, but the words were muttered, and inaudible to the observer sitting on one side of the bed. The sister, who stayed in the room, did not ask her to repeat her words, and Mrs Y did not herself do so. The room remained in silence for about a minute until the return of the doctor with the registrar she had gone to find. Sister then told the doctors she had found the head, 'up here', indicating a position at the side of the woman's abdomen. The doctor said 'Oh,' looking worried, and the registrar commented 'Fighting back, huh? We'll put a drip up and get the contractions going to move the head down.' He then left the room, and Mrs Y made a further inaudible remark, to which no one responded. Her legs were taken out of stirrups, Sister listened to the foetal heart, and the doctor started to comment on the drip, asking Mrs Y whether she had had one during the previous induction, and when she said no, telling her it was like a blood test, only worse. The professional comments then shifted to the technicalities of putting in a drip, encouraging noises from the doctor, a check that Mrs Y had never previously had a blood transfusion, and instructions from Sister about what to do if the drip alarm went off. This advice marked the end of the period of concentration on induction.

This short incident is a good illustration both of Mrs Y's style, and of the problems which bedevil teaching on the labour ward. Mrs Y, it will be recalled, was short of sleep. She was also in considerable discomfort during the period of the doctor's attempts to break her membranes; she could be seen clutching the side of the mattress. The staff told her to take deep breaths from time to time, and she was moving her feet in the stirrups in a way which suggested (and which the observer later confirmed by asking) that her legs were also in an awkward position. Further, a woman lying on her back with her feet in stirrups is not in the best position for self-assertion of any kind.

The doctor mainly involved had an easy conversational manner, and a particular style of talking through inductions, both as a means of providing information on what was going to happen and as a means of easing tension. She also made use of the fact that she *was* a woman doctor to try and reduce the potential embarrassment of this highly undignified position. On this occasion she, too, was short of sleep, and her patter was not as fluent as the observer had previously heard it; in addition, she had little verbal help from the sister who was providing practical aid. Nevertheless, as this incident shows, she did talk about what had gone wrong before she went for advice from the registrar. The mutters from Mrs Y suggest that, not surprisingly, she had not fully understood what was happening, but the staff did not pick up these mutters and deal with whatever problem they represented.

Further evidence emerged later of Mrs Y's wish for information. Once the drip was set up and various routine tasks completed (including the administration of magnesium trisilicate, without explanation), sister left the room, and the observer began her established routine of chatting to the patient, both to find out certain facts and, more important at this stage, to help the patient to accept her continued presence as non-intrusive. In the course of this sociable chatter, Mrs Y asked the observer what the drip did — 'Does it expand your waters?' Mrs Y clearly had informational needs in relation to induction which she had not managed to satisfy by relating to the staff responsible. Mrs Y developed a pattern of asking for information only from people with whom she had previously had some sociable conversation. A house officer, assigned to her care, had made an effort to chat while doing routine observations, and Mrs Y asked her 'Does it [the head] have to be right down before you break my waters?' The house officer explained that it was important to know first which way the baby was going to settle, to avoid finding the cord, or the baby's shoulder, coming first, and finished by saying 'It's not your problem anyway, 'cos you're alright and the baby's alright.' Mrs Y asked no more questions of the house officer.

At shift change at 1.00 p.m. a sister and a staff midwife took over responsibility for Mrs Y. The staff midwife was inexperienced but had apparently already developed a style which involved a lot of information-giving. She arrived with the trolley prepared for a further attempt at an ARM, and proceeded to explain the various implements; she had had no previous opportunity to chat to Mrs Y. She made it explicit that she was telling Mrs Y about the equipment to reassure her 'Otherwise you think — ooh!' Mrs Y responded by saying 'Yes, she did explain before . . . I think I'm past bothering now.'

Beyond Information – Towards Reassurance

Both Mrs X and Mrs Y reached a point where their need for information was not their only expressed need. Mrs X had been able to arrange for her needs to be met; Mrs Y seemed to have more difficulty in this respect, asking ineffective questions, or questions addressed to the 'wrong' people, at the beginning. Her comment that she was 'past bothering' may reflect her tiredness (for she had only dozed during the morning), her weariness of the staff's attempts to get her labour organised, her unfamiliarity with the midwife; it might also reflect the cut-off point noted by Korsch, Gozzi and Francis,[14] who found, in doctor-patient interviews, that after several ineffective attempts to obtain information, patients are likely to give up, and may not register information if it is finally given to them.

Informational needs did, however, appear to merge into other sorts of needs, and the magnesium trisilicate incident with Mrs X illustrates this clearly. The midwife who told her that feeling sick was a good sign did so in response to Mrs X's comment that she was not normally sick. She apparently interpreted Mrs X's remark as an oblique request for reassurance, and provided it; Mrs X, with no knowledge of 'normal' behaviour in labour, could quite reasonably be seen as looking for information on the norm against which she could judge her own progress. She raised similar issues when she mentioned that the baby was pressing on her right side, with some concern in her voice, and again was reassured 'He's a bigger lad than we thought', and also when she commented on the odd lump in the middle of her abdomen, which had appeared two to four weeks ago; the staff midwife laughed and patted the lump, and Mr X commented that the baby must have nowhere to put its feet. These oblique expressions of a need to be reassured that things were normal began at about 4.30 p.m., and the themes of the soreness on her right side, and the extra lump, did persist.

No further concerns of this kind emerged until near delivery. Mrs X's exceptional ability to control her urge to push misled the experienced staff midwife in charge of her case into believing that Mrs X was not yet ready to push. This misunderstanding led her to call in a doctor, because Mrs X was so long in second stage. The doctor did not speak to Mr and Mrs X, and after he had left Mrs X asked the staff midwife 'Who was that? He looked worried', and was told that he always looked like that; Mrs X was transferred to the delivery room and encouraged to push. Mrs X then reverted to her earlier pattern of asking questions, 'What can you see? What colour hair has it? I feel as if I'm going to burst – is that all right?' 'Is he all right?' The third question 'I feel as if

I'm going to burst' reflects the important issue of normality. Mrs X, in her first labour, could not know what was normal, but had the ability to express what she felt and to ask whether this was all right. The inevitable fourth question is also concerned with the normality issue.

Mrs Y's problems with normality were, of course, rather different from those of Mrs X. Her labour clearly did not begin normally; not only had she not started spontaneously, but the medical procedures were clearly abnormal as well. She also felt that the course of this labour was abnormal for her; at 6.37 p.m. came the first comment that she had not had so much pain with her first baby, and this combination of pain and worry became steadily more intense. 'I'll never make it.' 'I can't understand it, it's been so long.' 'I don't think I can stand it much longer', and at 8.40 p.m., to her husband, 'Why can't they just give me a Caesar and have done with it.' Her husband, trying to mediate between her and the staff, said at 8.00 p.m. 'It's just that she can't understand why she's had all this trouble, when she didn't with the other two.'

For Mrs Y, the problem as she expressed it was not just that she was in pain, but that she did not *expect* to be in so much pain. The staff's reassurances that she would in fact survive labour, and that she was progressing, were ineffective, and probably this is only what could be expected, particularly since the staff themselves were concerned about the persistent pain she was having, and turned the drip off to avoid the risk of a ruptured uterus. Although part of this problem is educational, teaching *on the ward* would be no solution. Mrs Y might have been less worried if she had earlier been helped to understand how different labours could be — but what she wanted most was pain relief, not an explanation of the variability of labour.

Towards Decision-Making

Information could be requested not only as an aid to peace of mind, but also as a basis for decision-making. Mrs X had hoped to be able to manage without pain relief; the length of her labour was therefore of considerable importance to her, not just to know how long she was going to have to cope with contractions, but also because she had to decide whether to try to cope without medication. In addition, she was knowledgeable enough about the different types of pain relief to be aware that the stage in labour she had reached should affect the decision on what to use. Her first 'How far on do you think I am?' came at 5.15 p.m., and 'How long' recurred increasingly, and more persistently, until the end of her last vaginal examination at 10.55 p.m.: 'How long?' 'Not long.' 'How long?' 'About half an hour.' The unwillingness of this staff midwife to give a time estimate was found to a greater or lesser degree in all those who cared for her; Mrs X did often manage to persuade people to give some estimate, or at least a milestone at which an estimate would be possible, like the next vaginal examination. Since her progress was slower than her various attendants estimated, this persistence did not necessarily meet her needs, but it did meet her desire for information.

On the basis of this information she tried gas and oxygen at about 6.00 p.m., found it not very helpful, and by 8.15 p.m., when the midwife she had become attached to was required elsewhere in the hospital, was finding the pains and the absence of 'her' midwife hard to bear, despite the presence of her husband. The sister substituting for 'her' midwife came in at 8.15 p.m. and asked 'Are you managing to cope?' Mrs X replied 'Just about — it is getting pretty bad.' Sister said 'I wonder if I should give you something?' 'It's a bit late now, isn't it?' 'I wouldn't give you a full dose.' 'I thought it took a while to work.' 'It does take a little while. Do you want to push?' 'It's pushing down now.' Sister felt her abdomen, watched the monitor, mentioned the weather, and then said 'Do you feel you want something a bit stronger than that?' 'Well, what would it be?' 'An injection, actually.' 'And how would it make me feel?' 'Drunk.' Mrs X had no enthusiasm for the injection, but said that the gas and oxygen made her feel sleepy; Sister told her that an injection would do this too, but relax her as well. She told the midwife, in response to a question, that she had wanted to manage without drugs. Her husband encouraged her to have something, to make it easier for herself; the sister told her nothing would harm the baby, that the injection would work 'in a few minutes', that in fact labour might be taking longer *because* she had had no sedation, since her own tension could be slowing the process down. When Mrs X still showed no enthusiasm for an injection, Sister suggested a stronger gas. At this point Mrs X appeared to give up, and asked Sister what she would recommend. Sister said that it was difficult at this stage, because Mrs X was so far on in labour; had she been in charge, Mrs X would have had an injection earlier. After a pause, during which Mrs X had a contraction, Sister said 'Shall I get you the gas, and you can try if it is a bit better than that one?' She went to find the Penthrane, and Mrs X used this until she reached the second stage.

This incident is revealing in a number of ways. Mrs X had been correctly informed about the effects of pethidine at antenatal classes. She knew that it took up to half an hour to take effect; she knew that it was not recommended in late first stage labour because of the risks to the baby.[15] She also seemed to be aware that it might make her feel

different and wanted more information on this point. She did not
seem to be familiar with Penthrane; observation of her previous experience with the gas and oxygen mask suggests that she had not been
taught how to use a mask in classes. She had, therefore, some relevant
information, and needed more to make any decision. The sister, however, provided her with information on pethidine which, to some
extent, contradicted in its implications what she had been told at
classes. Not surprisingly, Mrs X gave up the effort to make decisions
against a background of support for some form of pain relief from her
husband and the sister, and her increasing difficulty in coping with the
pain.

Mrs Y, it could be argued, was in a far worse position to make any
decisions at all. She had no training in self-help techniques, her husband
was absent for much of the time and had no previous training in how to
be useful, and she was coping with a labour which had abnormal
features, both from her point of view and from that of the staff. She
did not, however, despite her considerable pain, abandon all interest
in information related to decisions. After a vaginal examination at
7.30 p.m. the sister in charge, knowing that little progress had been
made, that Mrs Y had a swollen cervix, and that she was in considerable pain, suggested an epidural anaesthetic: 'Have you heard of an
epidural? It's an injection into your back, to take away the pain.' Mrs Y
asked 'How do you push, when . . .?' and Sister replied, 'We'll sort that
out later. I'm not promising anything, mind, but you would consider
it?' 'Yes, anything to stop the pain.' Mrs Y's query does in fact represent one of the major drawbacks of epidural anaesthetics, that they
can block out the urge to push. In the circumstances this was neither
the main concern of the sister nor of Mrs Y, but it is interesting that
she found the resources to ask; she also, after the first, ineffective
epidural had been put in, asked the staff nurse with the information-
giving style what it did.

The theoretical alternative to medication is self-help. Mrs X was
trained in NCT breathing techniques, and was visibly using these during
the period from about 7.45 p.m. to 8.35 p.m., when she was given
Penthrane; she used the gas and oxygen mask only intermittently. In
this she had help and support from her husband, who consulted the
NCT leaflets with her, encouraged her and timed contractions. This
last, according to Mrs X, was at the staff midwife's suggestion to see
how things were going, not for record purposes. The staff midwife
offered no other help, and did not seem to be aware that the couple
were NCT trained; she did not refer to the leaflets, which were not used

in her presence, though they were not hidden either.

Mrs Y had no training. She did, however, have problems with pain, and these were apparent to the staff at times when medication was not a practical answer. At 4.35 p.m. Mrs Y was given pethidine. The staff midwife then started routine checks, registered, but did not act on, Mrs Y's backache, registered her complaint that she felt sick and started to organise a glucose drip for her. Before this was done, Mrs Y was sick. The staff midwife also had problems with the monitor, which needed changing twice before 5.30 p.m., and registered the possibility that Mrs Y was fully dilated and ready to push. At 5.30 p.m. Sister did a vaginal examination to check on this. During this hour the pethidine could be expected to be starting to work, but was clearly not providing enough help for Mrs Y. As a supplement to pethidine, therefore, the staff midwife and Sister encouraged her to breathe deeply. Since this team of two had other patients to attend to as well as the list of problems with Mrs Y, it is not surprising that they were unable to encourage her very consistently. In addition, deep breathing as a technique for dealing with pain in labour is thought by a number of authorities to be ineffective, since it increases diaphragmatic pressure on the fundus during contractions.[16] It was not a technique encouraged by the hospital's physiotherapists, who were also responsible for teaching local community staff how to teach physical preparation.

Teaching on the Labour Ward

The foregoing description has focused on the expressed needs of the patients, rather than the problems of the staff. Some of these, like clinical complexity and pressure of time, are, however, obvious from the material. Others deserve more attention. For example, women's demands for information may be impossible to fulfil, not because of under-staffing, but because the staff cannot know the answer with any certainty. The cases of both Mrs X and Mrs Y show staff making judgements about how long labour will last, and being wrong. These members of staff were not inexperienced juniors. Women like Mrs X, who persist in asking for this information, *may* get an estimate which is accurate, but because labour is unpredictable this cannot be guaranteed. Similarly, requests for information which imply a wish for re-assurance that this phenomenon is normal represent a demand for reassurance that is, finally, impossible to meet. Donna Shields refers to 'the need to be assured of a safe outcome for mother and baby'.[17] Yet all that a midwife can honestly give is assurance that there is no reason why this should not be the case. Reassurance that this phenomenon,

whatever it is, is normal does not constitute reassurance that all will
continue to be normal. Those who argue against home confinements do
so from the position that no labour is normal except in retrospect. This
applies to hospital too.

Entirely satisfactory information, either for the making of decisions
or for reassurance, is not available to women in labour because it is not
available to midwives, or to doctors. This does not mean that information will cease to be sought, or given; it will continue to be used, by
women in labour and the midwives who care for them, to make the best
of a complicated situation. The problems concerned with the rate of
progress and normality of labour are probably the most difficult ones
involved in teaching about childbirth. They are also those which cannot
be tackled beforehand, except in very broad outline, because they relate
only to one individual labour. Either this sort of teaching is attempted
on the labour ward, or it will not be achieved at all. Because women
demand information, it is no solution to redefine these problems as
being problems of care, although good care is important too. An increased awareness of the likelihood that women may want information, will
increase the chances of staff meeting this type of need more successfully; an increased understanding on all sides that teaching does not
require, and midwives cannot give, final certainty would help the learning
process. Perfect matching of patient, teacher and setting may not be
possible in practice. But while there is a demand for teaching to solve
problems for women in labour, midwives have a responsibility to try to
meet it.

A Return to Practical Problems

Some efforts to meet these demands could be made within the existing
framework of hospital care. Staff could be more attuned to women's
needs for information, and more prepared to provide it. Mrs X's problems with information on pethidine, and even more clearly Mrs Y's
difficulties with her complicated early period on the labour ward, show
that staff do not always recognise poorly expressed requests for information, or react informatively to clear ones, even when they have the
time available to devote to this. Clearly there is room for improvement
here. Increased sensitivity on the part of the staff, however, would not
solve all the problems of teaching on the labour ward. Teaching self-
help methods requires both knowledge and time on the part of the staff;
it appears that neither of these requirements were met in the case of

Mrs Y. Courses on self-help methods for labour ward staff could help with the problem of knowledge, but not with the problem of time. Because labour ward staff may be expected to have at least one, if not both problems, women who go to childbirth classes are often encouraged to tell their husbands what they have learnt in classes, so that the men can take on the role of labour coach identified by Donna Shields as a useful part of care in labour.

It is at this point that the problems of teaching on the labour ward are shown to be insoluble within the existing framework of present staffing levels and almost 100 per cent hospital deliveries. If a woman is advised to take a helper with her, this is a sensible admission by hospital staff that they cannot provide the continuous caring presence of someone known to the patient. Where a woman is advised to see that her helper is trained to support her in using self-help techniques, if this is what she wishes to do, this again is a realistic admission that staffing levels and the unpredictable pattern of work on the labour ward preclude such support being *reliably* available from the staff. Solutions must therefore be sought outside the existing framework, and one of these is to call in outside people to support women in labour. Most such 'outsiders' are husbands, but some women may bring a relative or a friend. These are solutions found by the women themselves. Some experiments have been made with 'outsiders' who derive from the health service rather than from the private arrangements made by the women concerned; physiotherapists, for example, provide help during labour with self-help methods in some hospitals, though again there are too few staff available for this to be a possibility for every woman. Other experiments include the use of volunteers, who arrange to meet women who would like lay support in labour before they go into hospital, join them when they are admitted, and stay with them through their labour. Volunteers here represent substitutes for husbands, relatives or friends, available to women who have no one who would be willing to provide the support which such a person can give. If they are to provide help beyond that of a caring presence, they would need to be trained in self-help techniques, as a husband needs training if he is to support his wife in this way.

These solutions to the difficulties of midwives in teaching on the labour ward represent a willingness to accept that not all these difficulties will yield to increased staff sensitivity, or to courses for midwives in self-help methods. Solutions which rely on outside voluntary help have the merit of being cheap and, therefore, comparatively practical. It is worth briefly considering other solutions which are probably more radical, certainly more expensive, and therefore apparently less practical, but which also involve a recognition of the limitations of improving practice within the existing framework. One such solution is, of course, a considerable improvement in staffing levels. If midwives cannot provide the teaching which is a part of good midwifery care, then, the argument would run, there should be a lot more midwives. An alternative radical solution is to reject the existing shape of the problem. If the need for teaching on the labour ward is in part related to unfamiliarity with hospital routine, procedures, equipment and staff, then why not reduce the size and scope of the problem by drastically reducing the number of women delivered in hospital?[18] At home a woman would be in a familiar environment, and could reasonably hope to be attended by a community midwife who had cared for her in pregnancy. The reduction in the number of hospital deliveries could also give hospital staff more time to devote to high risk women who were selected for hospital care.

Both these more radical solutions raise further problems, on issues beyond the scope of this book. They are advanced, in outline only, as a means of stressing the point that satisfactory solutions to the difficulties of midwives in carrying out their teaching role on the labour ward are not available within the existing framework. Calling in outsiders is one possibility; greatly increasing the number of midwives is another; reorganising the maternity services is a third. Useful improvements could be made by encouraging staff to be more aware of women's needs for information, and how staff can best meet them, and by seeing that labour ward staff are conversant with modern self-help techniques. Such improvements would be worth making; it would, however, be of no service to staff or patients to pretend that they will completely solve the problems of teaching and learning on the labour ward.

Notes

1. Grantly Dick Read, *Natural Childbirth* (Heinemann, London, 1933).

2. D. Haire, 'The Cultural Warping of Childbirth', *ICEA News Special Issue* (Washington, 1972).

3. Jane R. Gillett, 'Helping Those Who Have Not Been to Preparation for Childbirth Classes', *Midwives' Chronicle and Nursing Notes* (February 1977), pp. 32-3. Here she explicitly recants contrary views expressed in an earlier article.

4. The figure of 45 per cent is compounded from the results of various studies: G. Chamberlain, 'Antenatal Education', *Midwife, Health Visitor and Community Nurse*, vol. 11 (September 1975), p. 289; Elizabeth R. Perkins, 'The Pattern of Women's Attendance at Antenatal Classes: Is This Good Enough?', *Health Education Journal* (1980, in press); N.J. Spencer, 'The Identification and Management of

Illness by Parents of Young Children', unpublished MPhil thesis, University of Nottingham, 1980. B.M. Hibbard *et al.* in 'The Effectiveness of Antenatal Education', *Health Education Journal*, vol. 38, no. 2 (1979), pp. 39-46, classified only 28 per cent of their sample of primigravadae as attenders, but their definition of attendance required women to go to at least 75 per cent of mothercraft classes; thus the figures are not comparable.

5. Elizabeth R. Perkins, 'And Did You Go to Classes, Mrs Brown?', *Midwives' Chronicle and Nursing Notes* (December 1979), pp. 422-5.

6. For views of women connected with voluntary organisations, or in other ways not necessarily representative of the total population, see: Sheila Kitzinger, *The Good Birth Guide* (Fontana, Glasgow, 1979); John and Jean Lennane, *Hard Labour* (Gollancz, London, 1974). For research studies, see Ann Cartwright, *Human Relations and Hospital Care* (Routledge & Kegan Paul, London, 1964); Hazel Houghton, 'Problems of Hospital Communication' in Gordon McLachlan (ed.), *Problems and Progress in Medical Care: Essays on Current Research*, 3rd series (Oxford University Press, London, 1968).

7. For psychological interpretations of this variation, see: Helene Deutsch, *The Psychology of Women: A Psychoanalytic Interpretation, Motherhood*, vol. 2 (Research Books, London, 1947); and Leon Chertok, *Motherhood and Personality, Psychosomatic Aspects of Childbirth*, English edition (Tavistock, London, 1969).

8. Elizabeth R. Perkins, 'Having a Baby: An Educational Experience?', Occasional Paper 6 (Leverhulme Health Education Project, University of Nottingham, 1978).

9. See the review of the literature in Debra L. Roter, 'Patient Participation in the Patient-provider Interaction: The Effects of Patient Question Asking on the Quality of Interaction, Satisfaction and Compliance', *Health Education Monographs* (Winter, 1977), p. 281.

10. Donna Shields, 'Nursing Care in Labour and Patient Satisfaction: A Descriptive Study', *Journal of Advanced Nursing*, vol. 3 (1978), pp. 535-50.

11. For a discussion of different types of need, see J.S. Bradshaw, 'A Taxonomy of Social Need' in Gordon McLachlan (ed.), *Problems and Progress in Medical Care: Essays on Current Research*, 7th series (Oxford University Press, London, 1972).

12. For introductory discussion of method in observation studies, see: Jill Macleod Clark and Lisbeth Hockey, *Research for Nursing: A Guide for the Enquiring Nurse* (HM & M Publishers, Aylesbury, 1979); Leonard Schatzman and Anselm L. Strauss, *Field Research: Strategies for a Natural Sociology* (Prentice Hall, Englewood Cliffs, New Jersey, 1973); Open University Course DE304 *Research Methods in Education and the Social Sciences*, 1978. For studies based on observation method, see Howard S. Becker, Blanche Everett, G. Hughes and Anselm L. Strauss, *Boys in White: Student Culture in Medical School* (Chicago University Press, Chicago, 1961); David Sudnow, *Passing On: The Social Organisation of Dying* (Prentice Hall, Englewood Cliffs, New Jersey, 1967); Nancy Stoller Shaw, *Forced Labour: Maternity Care in the United States* (Pergamon, Oxford, 1974).

13. During the winter of 1978-9, the observer sat with three women in Unit A, and seven in Unit B, during part or all of their labours, and observed admissions of one further woman in Unit A and three in Unit B. She spent approximately 24 hours observing labour in Unit A, over a period of three working days. These periods were not consecutive, and she also spent a number of 'blank' days at Unit B, waiting to see whether there would be any patients for the particular consultant whose permission she had obtained for observation, and furthering her understanding of the working of the units. She spent her blank days at Unit B in the

midwives' duty room, used mainly by sisters, or at the midwives' station, and thus had the chance to ask and answer questions without disrupting the work of the staff.

14. B.M. Korsch, E.M. Gozzi and V. Francis, 'Gaps in Doctor-patient Communication', *Pediatrics*, vol. 42, no. 5 (November 1968), pp. 855-71.

15. Michael Rosen, 'Pain and its Relief' in Tim Chard and Martin Richards (eds.), *Benefits and Hazards of the New Obstetrics: Clinics in Developmental Medicine*, no. 64 (Heinemann in association with Spastics International Medical Publications, London, 1977).

16. See the discussion in M. Williams and D. Booth, *Antenatal Education: Guidelines for Teachers* (Churchill Livingstone, Edinburgh, 1974).

17. Shields, 'Nursing Care in Labour and Patient Satisfaction: A Descriptive Study'.

18. Sheila Kitzinger and John Davis (eds.), *The Place of Birth* (Oxford University Press, Oxford, 1978).

3 TEACHING ABOUT LABOUR: THE CONTRIBUTION OF ANTENATAL CLASSES

The Problem of Expectations

For most women expecting their first baby, the phenomenon of birth is nowadays a process completely outside their experience. When women routinely had their babies at home, friends and neighbours and younger children might be present during part of labour, or even for the birth. The concentration of births in hospital means that a few women now witness another woman's labour, unless they are professionally involved. Their expectations of their own labour are thus theoretical, rather than based on observation. Antenatal classes attempt to provide information and techniques which can relate expectations to reality; they do not, however, operate in a vacuum. On the contrary, women attending classes in late pregnancy will have absorbed a variety of information or misinformation, frequently characterised by antenatal teachers as 'old wives' tales' — or 'new wives' tales'.

The content of these tales varies, but the expectations to which they give rise can be characterised by three types. The first is the 'old wives' tale' *par excellence*: 'in sorrow thou shalt bring forth children'. Labour is long hours of agonising pain, accompanied by straining on knotted sheets tied to bedposts. There is blood, sweat and tears in abundance; the fear of death, or injury, for mother or baby or both, is ever present. A contrasting version is the 'new wives' tale' — babies are born between nine and five o'clock in antiseptic modern hospitals where doctors hover in attendance to see that the process goes according to medically approved criteria. This pattern is two-faced. Some women see medical control as a guarantee that mother will suffer no pain and baby no deformity. Others fear that the hospital will make of labour an alienating experience where machines matter and people do not. A third pattern of expectation might be called the 'free spirit's tale'. Childbirth is ecstasy, providing the doctors will leave you alone. Working in harmony with your contractions, you and your partner will achieve a peak experience as you push the baby out.

All these experiences are possible, though bedposts are in short supply these days. None of them is guaranteed; perhaps none of them is even probable. Women who go into labour firmly attached to any of these concepts are ill-equipped to cope with their own individual

45

pattern of labour. The woman who believes labour is agony or that
hospital staff are inhuman may make matters worse by her fear and
tension or aggression. The woman looking forward to the joys of technological childbirth or the peak experience may be disappointed by
the technology, her attendants or her own body's reactions. Antenatal
classes have the difficult task of relating to reality women's existing
expectations (and each woman may half believe in more than one of
the 'tales' of labour). Ann Oakley, in her study of first-time mothers,[1]
found that 93 per cent of her sample said that birth was different from
what they had expected. The task of antenatal teachers is not made
easier by the tremendous variability of labour, and the practical impos-
sibility of predicting its course for any one woman.

The Collection of Data

To see how different antenatal teachers approached this common problem, a participant observation study was undertaken,[2] involving attendance at three different antenatal courses: a health service course
arranged in a hospital maternity unit, another at a health centre in a
small town, and a National Childbirth Trust course[3] in a larger town
held in the teacher's own home. All courses had eight sessions; the
observer attended seven of the eight evening NCT classes, the same
number of afternoon sessions at the health centre, and all eight hospital
sessions, though she was unable to attend the two evening sessions for
both parents held at the hospital, or the visit of the health centre class
to the hospital where the women were to be confined.

A variety of personnel was involved in teaching these courses: two
obstetric physiotherapists and two midwifery sisters at the hospital class,
alternating to cover holidays, together with five pupil midwives; two
health visitors (one acting as a relief only) and a midwife at the health
centre class; and an NCT trained antenatal teacher who was both a
mother of three children and a practising obstetric physiotherapist. All
the staff regularly involved were aware of the observer's status, though
it was not always possible for the observer to introduce herself to the
different pupil midwives before the session. The observer, a married
woman in her late twenties, made no attempt to pass as pregnant with
the expectant mothers, though she usually wore fairly loose clothing,
and with many of the women her non-pregnant state became a running
joke. At the NCT reunion after the babies were born she was rather
surprised to be asked quite seriously where her baby was — the

questioner had been an irregular attender and had assumed that the observer was in early pregnancy! No other woman, to the observer's knowledge, misunderstood her position.

The observer acted as a member of the class wherever possible, usually waiting in waiting rooms with the rest for the NHS classes to start, and trying to avoid being singled out for special treatment during the class. She did not use a notebook during the sessions — it is impossible to practise the best position for pushing a baby out and make notes at the same time! — but wrote up her observations as soon as possible after the class finished, and certainly the same day. The expectant mothers were not apparently inhibited by the observer's presence; they accepted her as a member of the group, though a rather deviant one. This was also true of most of the teachers, with the exception of the health visitor, who emphasised the observer's professional status.

Physiology and Pain

Bringing expectations into line with probabilities can begin with basic facts — the physiology of labour and delivery. All courses recognised this as important; the community course in the health centre spent part of one session talking about labour, part of a further session revising it, and part of the last session attempting to integrate the relaxation method, hitherto not related to labour, with the progress of the woman in labour through first and second stage. The hospital course devoted part of a midwives' session to talking about labour, and the physiotherapist integrated her physical preparation with descriptions of the stages at which, for example, particular breathing patterns were appropriate. The National Childbirth Trust course followed the same pattern as shown by the hospital physiotherapist, integrating the practice of breathing levels or relaxation with the theory of normal childbirth. Both used the device of a labour rehearsal, which enables women to practise their techniques in the order in which they are likely to be needed; the health centre course included material in its last session which could have been used in this way, but it was taught out of order, with second stage techniques sandwiched between first stage ones.

A realistic expectation for pregnant women in Britain is that they will push their baby out. All the tutors made this explicit, and the hospital and NCT classes practised the position for pushing; women attending these courses were told that they would push most efficiently sitting up, and that plenty of pillows, or a husband's arm round them, or

both, would be a help. The community class tutor did not ask her class
to practise the correct position for pushing, 'in case it starts you off',
and did not mention the virtues of sitting up. All women were taught
about the panting breathing which can help a woman to resist the urge
to push as the baby's head is born.

The physiology of labour, necessary though it is as a basis for further
learning, is not much immediate help in tackling the problems of expectations outlined earlier. Physiology cannot answer the question 'How
will I feel?' Pain figures in all three of our patterns of expectation. The
'old wives' tale' has it as a dominant feature; the 'new wives' tale' relies
on medical technology to abolish it. The 'free spirit's tale' abolishes
pain by redefining it as a new, overpowering sensation, and incorpor-
ating techniques to work with it, not against it. In this sense, para-
doxically, this romantic view of childbirth is the most practical one, in
that the woman has something she can do to help fulfil her expectations; in technological childbirth she must rely on her attendants to
do it. Childbirth classes include material on self-help and medical help
with pain. The balance of emphasis and the relationship between the
two, however, vary; so does the picture of labour presented to
pregnant women.

Self-Help with Pain

Self-help methods vary, but they rely on two main principles: relaxation, so that tension does not obstruct the work of the uterus, and
breathing techniques, which can function either as distraction from
pain or as adaptation to the work of the uterus, or both. The community class relied almost exclusively on relaxation, tackling breathing
techniques for labour only during the last session of the eight week
course. The hospital class and the National Childbirth Trust teacher
taught relaxation at the beginning of the course and incorporated short
relaxation periods into the rest of their teaching. Breathing techniques
and relaxation were thus practised together, as they were intended to
be used.

The relaxation techniques employed relied on different basic principles. The hospital physiotherapist and the NCT teacher, also a physiotherapist, both used the Mitchell method of relaxation, the deliberate
contraction of different muscle groups followed by their relaxation.
The women practising this method are enabled to feel the difference
between a tense and relaxed muscle very quickly, and are also provided

with a way of checking for tension and correcting it. The NCT teacher
also taught dissociative relaxation, tensing one muscle and relaxing the
rest, as preparation for labour when the uterus is working and the rest
of the body should be relaxed. The health visitor used a script written
by a physiotherapist for use in the community, based on the psycho-
physical method.[4] This used imagery associated with relaxation to
induce a relaxed mind and a relaxed body. The women lay on camp
beds for relaxation and the health visitor tried to arrange a restful
room, with, for example, the curtains half drawn. She used her own
voice to achieve a soothing effect. This method relies in part on the
practitioner and her students being in agreement about what is a
relaxing image. The script used by this particular health visitor incorporated the suggestions of swelling joints (which could be associated
with arthritis), head hanging back uncontrollably, and eyeballs rolling
upwards (which could be associated with death) and, as one woman
explained the method, 'Imagine water is running up one arm and down
the other and you have to breathe through your fingers and, I mean,
while you are doing it there you are laughing.'[5] It may be difficult to
use this particular method, which relies on mental influence on physical tension, without suggesting images at all.

The effect of the two methods on the subject is not the same; the
community method has many affinities with Benson's[6] basic relaxation method, derived from his work on transcendental meditation and
its effects on high blood pressure. He advises a quiet room, an unpres-
sured approach, a comfortable position and either closed eyes or a fixed
gaze. He suggests concentration on one particular word in conjunction
with deliberate breathing, whereas the community method emphasises
deep breathing only. Benson distinguishes the 'relaxation response'
(with the physical characteristics of lower blood pressure, slower pulse,
and reduced oxygen consumption) from sleep, though pointing out that
using basic relaxation techniques while lying down can readily induce
sleep. The community class who practised relaxation lying down, under
the health visitor's guidance, included women who regularly went to
sleep. This caused no concern to the health visitor; it did, however,
create difficulties for the women when they tried to practise at home,
since they did not know what most of the relaxation pattern was.
Either they went to sleep again, or they did not relax.

The 'relaxation response' can be achieved most readily by the inexperienced in a quiet room, but with practice can be induced anywhere. Pregnant women will later need to use relaxation in an unfamiliar labour ward which may well be noisy. While the health visitor stres-

sed the importance of practice at home, she did not try to encourage
the practice of this skill in a less favourable setting. Another problem
for the use of this method in labour in hospital is the reaction of a
number of women in the class to the process of *emerging* from the
relaxed state — they found the feeling of 'coming round' unpleasant.
This could create difficulties for them if they were expected to respond
reasonably quickly to requests from hospital staff.

The relationship between community relaxation techniques and the
'relaxation response' suggests that most women will find the community
method pleasant, providing they do not react badly to the imagery
used. The context in which they learn it involves them in the minimum
of effort, since the soothing, repetitive voice of the tutor has an additional relaxing effect. Where this is used as the main element of preparation for labour, it may encourage expectations corresponding to the
'free spirit's tale' — relax and enjoy it. Such expectations may be unrealistic. To quote again the woman who thought the relaxation
method was funny: 'I think they could explain the birth better, 'cos
how they've told you, you know, you just cough and drop it.'

The Mitchell method, on the other hand, relies on physical means of
inducing relaxation, rather than mental ones. The mind of the subject
can remain alert and aware of what is going on, while the body is
relaxed. When one woman went to sleep in the hospital class, on a very
hot day, the physiotherapist in charge was most concerned that she had
produced an unplanned and undesirable result. The Mitchell method
was taught in conjunction with breathing techniques for labour, as
distinct from breathing techniques for relaxation. The hospital course
distinguished different types of breathing, using descriptive labels
('tummy breathing'); the NCT course used a more elaborate but basic-
ally similar system, using letters as labels ('level A breathing'). The
implication of either system is that in labour, the woman is expected
to do something specific, not just lie back and enjoy it.

Lay and Medical Help

Many hospitals now allow husbands to join their wives in labour, and
some encourage them to be present. A husband is a potential source of
unskilled lay help. Antenatal classes may structure a woman's expectation of what her husband can do to help; they may encourage her to
turn him into a practised helper beforehand; they may even attempt to
provide tuition for husbands themselves. Whether they do so depends

partly on the tutor's attitude towards husbands, but also on the method taught. The health visitor, for example, was in favour of husbands being there for the birth because 'it's good for the whole family', but she made no suggestion that they might be useful. Since relaxation was almost all the physical preparation she taught, and the method relied heavily on mind over matter, this is perhaps not surprising. Both the hospital physiotherapist and the NCT teacher encouraged women to tell their husbands about the breathing techniques, to ask them to help with practice at home, and to teach the men how to rub their backs and how to prop them up in second stage labour. A fathers' night was arranged in both classes for the men to be taught directly.

The courses handled the issue of medical help differently in two respects: what women were told and what relationship medical help had to self-help. In the community classes, the function of relaxation was explained at the beginning as making it possible to avoid tightening the birth canal, so that the baby can be born easily, with less pain and more quickly. In the same session one particular type of pain relief was mentioned as a supplement to relaxation, and the group was told that a demonstration of the machine which delivered it would be available later. A more detailed description of the role of relaxation in labour was provided in the last class.

The demonstration of the Entonox machine took place during the fourth class. 'Entonox' is a mixture of nitrous oxide and oxygen, commonly referred to as 'gas and oxygen'. Because it contains more oxygen than ordinary air it is harmless, and it is one of a number of pain relieving drugs which are inhaled through a mask. The teacher demonstrating the use of the mask was a community midwife, new to the class, who told the group she was tired, and sounded cross. Almost all the group had trouble using the machine, and were told 'You'll all use it in labour, never fear.' She was very brisk with everyone, including one woman showing clear fear of the mask, and was inclined to put her arm round women's shoulders and hold the mask down on their faces. This may well be an entirely appropriate response to a woman who is panicking in late first stage labour. Force is not, however, generally recommended as a *teaching* technique. When staff are tired, they are likely to make mistakes — and the mistakes they make will reflect the professional instincts they have developed. This midwife appeared to have reverted to a pattern of action based on practical work on the labour ward, not on teaching.

She went on to talk about when the machine might be used, in late first stage labour. She had apparently not been briefed on the ground previously covered, and her vocabulary assumed a knowledge the group probably did not possess. She said, incorrectly,[7] that Entonox should not be combined with other drugs, and was voluble about the misguided behaviour of hospital staff who used combinations of drugs, thus knocking out the baby and the labour, and setting the whole process back. She said that gas and oxygen could be used only with permission,[8] and the general tenor of her talk and demonstration was that it was midwife-controlled rather than self-administered. No detail on other drugs was given. During a later session of the course one woman asked the health visitor whether epidural anaesthetics were available at the hospital where she was booked. The health visitor said she did not know, but expected that 'they' would do an epidural if the woman asked. There was no epidural service available at this hospital, since the provision of epidural anaesthesia is only possible when an anaesthetist can be present on the ward, or on call, during the whole of the period when it is used. This was not possible at the hospital concerned, and a woman wanting an epidural would have had to arrange transfer to a hospital where staffing was adequate to provide such a service.

This course provided no clear picture of the range of drugs available, and a medically-controlled view of what drugs were mentioned. The midwife's picture of labour as being grim enough to force women to use a mask they found unpleasant or frightening, contrasted sharply with the picture of easy labour conveyed through relaxation. The health visitor's statement that gas and oxygen was there as a supplement to relaxation was an explicit though frail link between the two.

The hospital course, divided evenly in time between midwives and physiotherapists, provided a clearer illustration of conflicting conceptions. The midwives' attitude to self-help seemed to vary between different midwives. The pupil who explained the process of labour encouraged breathing as a 'good thing'. Pain relief was left to another pupil, in a later session. This pupil was extremely nervous, and was rescued regularly by the sister in charge. These two appeared to have different approaches to the session, the pupil providing a technical account of the drugs available, and the sister in addition expressing her opinion of the advantages of drug use. The pupil explained the existence and effects of pethidine 'like feeling drunk — like looking down on yourself' and also explained about Entonox. This was offered for people to try as the session went on, the sister in charge trying it first. The staff explicitly recognised that some women were afraid of masks, and pointed out that one of the virtues of this method was that you could control it yourself, unlike the dentist's mask. No pressure was put on individuals to try it, and as people volunteered they were helped to use it while the conversation went on; in this way no public failures were created. In addition, two additional, stronger gases were mentioned, 'for women who get a little bit uncontrollable', according to sister; she also referred to a sleeping pill, for use during slow labour to give women a rest. Epidurals were mentioned as not being available because of the shortage of anaesthetists, and their disadvantages in blocking out the urge to push were also mentioned.

Women asked questions reflecting worries about lack of pain relief; for example, one commented 'I suppose you've just got to suffer.' Others were concerned about too much pain relief. Sister dealt promptly with the first anxiety: 'No one suffers in this hospital', but none of the midwives appeared to recognise the second. Questions about who decided when women were given drugs were answered in terms of midwives' discretion, related to vaginal examinations to determine progress. Sister had earlier said the women could use self-help, but also stated, during both pupils' sessions, that she saw no point in drug-free labour — 'We give no medals for a stiff upper lip.' She also made the point, originally in connection with enemas, but subsequently generalised, that the staff could not force a woman to do anything she did not want to do.

The midwives' composite approach to pain in labour was characterised by contradictions and partial explanations. The impression left by the lecture on the physiology of labour was, to quote the observer's field notes, that 'labour hurts, but we'll drug you and you won't remember it'. It was admitted that some women preferred to do without drugs, but they were clearly seen as eccentric; no side effects which might justify this stand were mentioned. The right to choose not to have drugs was acknowledged. In the instance observed, however, the question of who decides when to have what was dodged, although if women accept that drugs are desirable, this is clearly the next important question. The provision of clear information on the different drugs available and their possible effects, and the sensitive handling of the demonstration of Entonox, was undermined by the failure to confront the issue of who decides, and when. This is finally a matter for negotiation between the experienced midwife and the individual woman in labour,[9] but it would be possible to provide some guidance beforehand on the factors involved in making the decision: individual rate and stage of progress, and the characteristics of drugs, for example. The statement that 'nobody suffers in this hospital' is not an adequate answer to a complex question.

The physiotherapist's approach to pain in labour was more clearly articulated, and to some extent filled the gap left by the failure of the midwives to answer this question. She shared their basic perspective that labour hurts, introducing her part of the first session by saying that she was going to teach the group 'how to make yourself less uncomfortable'. She said that there were several techniques of relaxation, but 'this one will give you independence'. She made links between her methods and the medical help available, saying that women could certainly refuse pain relief if they wished to, but it would be wise not to make the refusal final; instead, she suggested that they said 'Ask me again in half an hour.' She also pointed out that pethidine would probably be refused towards the end of the first stage to avoid having a sedated mother who could not push very effectively; gas and oxygen could be used instead.

The National Childbirth Trust teacher, working alone except for one visit from a NCT breast feeding counsellor, was able to present a unitary picture of labour and delivery. She said clearly in the first session that the NCT did not promise painless labour; the methods she was teaching would help a woman to raise her pain threshold, not abolish pain altogether. She suggested that women should politely convey to the hospital staff that they would ask for pain relief if they wanted it. The different types of pain relief were discussed; she pointed out that the effects of pethidine varied from woman to woman, and that women could ask for half a dose first, to see how they reacted.[10] The London teaching hospital which she was attending to gain her obstetric physiotherapist's qualification gave the half dose routinely, but in the provinces, she said, it was necessary to ask for this. Epidural anaesthesia was also variable in its effects, since only 80 per cent of epidurals worked.[11] She felt that NHS classes were inclined to mislead women on the risk of needing a forceps delivery because of the epidural. The dominant impression given was that medical pain relief was an addition to the woman's own self-help methods, which she could use or not depending on how she got on in labour. In the case of complications, women could expect a pudendal block for a forceps delivery, and a caesarean operation might be done under epidural rather than general anaesthetic if the mother wanted this and the obstetrician felt it was practical.

Professional staff have been known to criticise the National Childbirth Trust for giving women expectations of labour which correspond to the 'free spirit's tale', and leaving midwives on the labour and postnatal wards to pick up the pieces when labour turns out to hurt after all. This criticism neglects the possibility that women will have expectations before they go to classes and may select classes which they think will enable them to fulfil their dreams. Certainly this is not a valid criticism of the teaching provided in this particular NCT class; indeed, if any class could be accused of making labour seem too easy, it would be the community class.

Coping with Hospital

Hospital is the preoccupation of the 'new wives' tale' and the 'free spirit's tale'. Those who believe in the inevitable benevolence of medical control may assume that their every need will be anticipated, and that what they are not offered they may not have, from drinks of water to injections; anything that does go wrong may be even more shattering because of their faith in the power of the doctor. Those who believe that much of obstetrics is better described in the old-fashioned phrase 'meddlesome midwifery' may feel that they have to fight the institution every step of the way to retain any hope of giving birth with dignity. For most first-time mothers, the hospital, the staff they will meet, and its procedures are likely to be as unknown as the sensations of labour.

Many courses now include a trip round the maternity unit; both the community and hospital classes did this, and the NCT teacher encouraged her students to go round the hospital where they were booked. In itself, this is useful; one mother in the hospital class said that her trip round the labour ward took away 'the terror of going into hospital'. It provides a clearer picture of the place of labour and delivery, and as such contributes to realistic expectations; fantasy about giving birth now has a context. In addition, direct teaching can give information on life in hospital. One issue, of course, is who will be there to take care of the woman in labour; one woman in the hospital class was naive enough to ask whether the consultant, who she had not yet seen, 'made his big entrance' at this point! The midwife made it clear that doctors were expected only in case of complications. The pupil midwife who taught the physiology of labour said that they liked to have husbands on the ward, because the staff could not be with every woman all the time, and it was good to have company; the health visitor, teaching a community class feeding that hospital, said to her group 'You won't be left alone.' Her lack of familiarity with hospital practice was noted earlier in the context of the epidural service.

The crucial relationship between preparation for hospital and expectations, however, lies in the degree to which women believe they will need to assert themselves. Both hospital and community midwives' attitude to this issue has already been discussed in the context of pain relief; further examples were noted in the hospital class in the neutral area of drinks. One woman said that she found plain water unpleasant to drink, and could she bring fruit juice instead; sister snapped 'You'd have to bring it in, we don't supply that.'[12] The midwife talking about the period immediately after the birth began her talk by telling the women that they would be given a cup of tea; over half an hour later one of the more outgoing and confident members of the class suddenly blurted out that tea made her feel sick. The midwife understandably looked surprised, and said that in that case she should ask for coffee instead. Both incidents illustrate a lack of explicit recognition of patient choice, even in minor matters. Expectations of being in hospital are likely to include the restriction of activity, and these midwives' handling of the issue of choice would confirm this.

The physiotherapist made a deliberate effort to encourage women to exercise choice in the areas where this was possible. She told her class that if they had backache, they could ask for one of the pillows in use in class — 'Just ask them for one of those pillows the physios use.' She pointed out that there was no need to lie on your back all the time just because the midwives examined you on your back; it was quite all right to move, and to ask for more pillows if you needed propping up. If there was a shortage, existing ones could be doubled up. Midwives, she pointed out, want you to be comfortable, because it is more efficient! As we saw earlier, she also modelled for the group a way of refusing drugs while keeping options open. The physiotherapist had the knowledge to be able to provide this encouragement and detailed examples of what it was perfectly all right to do. The health visitor was in a similar structural position to the physiotherapist, preparing women for labour, but not a member of the professional group supervising labour. In theory, therefore, she could have taken up a similar role; in practice, she chose to encourage women to put their faith in the hospital staff who would look after them. In view of her lack of information about the workings of the hospital where women in her class were booked for delivery, this may in fact have been her only option.

This need not necessarily be true of all who work in the community. The NCT teacher was preparing women for any of the four maternity units within her area, clearly a more difficult task than preparing for one. While she had her own professional experience and contacts, she also used the NCT system of labour reports, where women write about their labour, and reunions where they come back to meet the other women again, admire one another's babies, and talk about their experiences. She too encouraged women to ask for pillows, and for bedsocks if necessary in late first stage; she suggested husbands got organised with wet flannels to mop their wife's face, and small natural sponges for them to suck, and also suggested that they should ask whether there was any ice available. She too encouraged movement, this time both in and out of bed, saying there was no need to stay in bed in normal labour. She did, however, emphasise that once a woman's membranes had ruptured, she should go into hospital, and would then be expected to stay in bed to avoid the risk of a prolapsed cord. She stressed that pushing in second stage was most efficient if the woman was upright rather than flat, and suggested that women should if necessary ask to be delivered half sitting, and that husbands should organise pillows and prop their wives up.

This teacher's approach definitely favoured self-assertion — but politely. One of the group, expecting her fourth baby, commented: 'If you're nice to the staff, they'll be nice to you, by and large.'

Individual Variation

Labour is individual and unpredictable, outside very broad limits. Teaching about labour may give the impression that individuality is encouraged, or that it is suppressed. The recognition of individuality facilitates good teaching and good supportive care from the teacher to members of the group, but in the case of NHS classes it may also influence expectations of hospital care.

The health visitor and the midwives in the community and hospital groups made little effort to get to know the women they taught. The community midwife, visiting the community group once only, did look for women who were her particular responsibility, but did not identify the very tentative murmur from a woman she had not yet met. The health visitor used first names for the women (there were eight at the start of the course) but frequently forgot whether they had had babies before, and where they were booked for confinement. The hospital midwives called the register at the beginning of each class, 'Mrs —' and did not use names during the teaching sessions. This group started with 19 women. The physiotherapist did not learn names either, but her care of the women was more personal. She noticed when they found positions uncomfortable, and helped them to find alternatives, with pillows where necessary. She made it clear that she was willing to talk to husbands outside the official 'fathers' night' if they could not come because of shift work.

In extreme cases a failure to recognise personal variation can lose customers, for classes if not for the hospital. One woman attending the NCT class did so because of her experiences at the community class she had previously attended. She was a teacher, the only one in the community class to ask questions. She said that the health visitor in charge of this class had embarked on a criticism of the NCT, saying that she knew a teacher who had been to their classes and had found labour no easier as a result; had progressed from this to a comment that teachers and nurses made the worst patients, because they knew it all and were forever asking questions; and went on to ask if there were any teachers present. At this point the teacher decided that the NHS class had nothing to offer her, and joined the NCT class instead.

Personal variation is relevant not only to the handling of the class, which may raise expectations about the extent of individual choice permitted in hospital; it is also relevant to labour. Both the physiotherapist in the hospital class and the NCT teacher emphasised the extent of variation in labour. The physiotherapist said that women all reacted differently, and some felt more pain than others; it was impossible to describe how they would feel. The NCT teacher said that the only common factor in labour was difficulty in breathing; pain could be felt in back, legs or abdomen, and did not always come in contractions, but could be felt as a continuous ache. The health visitor placed less stress on variability, commenting that some women did have a painless first stage of labour, but not developing this theme. The issue did not arise in either hospital or community midwives' work, which is in keeping with the attitude displayed to issues of personal choice.

Individual variation continues beyond labour to delivery. Some women may have peak experiences at delivery; no class explicitly held out this hope. Others will have the reverse: a complicated delivery, a handicapped child, or even a stillbirth. Many more will fear that one or more of these may happen.[13] The hospital and community classes teachers did not comment on the possibility of problems, with the exception of induction, mentioned at the hospital class, which was said to be only used when the baby was overdue. None of the women raised this sort of question. The NCT teacher did discuss coping with complications in labour; she made extensive use of the presence of a mother who had been induced in her previous pregnancy, asking her to talk about her labour; she talked about forceps deliveries, telling women that they would probably be expected to work with the doctor, pushing and panting as instructed, in a similar way to a normal delivery. The possibility of caesarean section under epidural anaesthetic was mentioned here. She moved on from this to touch on handicap and stillbirth. She said that the hospital staff would give a mother the baby immediately after birth, if she asked, and this was probably the best time to see it, because the rush of energy after the birth would give extra resources to cope with the shock. The alternative of being left to worry was probably worse, even with a stillbirth. No member of the group took up the topic, but the opportunity was there.

The Effect of Professional Status on Teaching

British preparation for childbirth has been strongly influenced by the obstetrician Grantly Dick Read. He argued that a vicious circle of fear-tension-pain made labour and delivery more difficult than they need be, and attempted to break it in his own clinical practice by freeing women from the fear of childbirth.[14] To this end he used not only the techniques which have now been developed and extended to form modern physical preparation, but also the force of his own personality, encouraging his patients to believe that he would neither let them suffer nor engage in that generation's version of 'meddlesome midwifery', the over-enthusiastic use of forceps. Present day antenatal teachers lack some of Grantly Dick Read's advantages. They are unlikely to be present at the delivery of the women they teach, let alone in sole charge of it; physiotherapists, some health visitors and most voluntary childbirth teachers are not qualified to deliver babies even if their presence at the birth could be arranged. Thus they will, in most cases, have no opportunity to become a Svengali figure, or, more modestly, to support the women they teach during labour and encourage them to use the techniques they have learnt. This means that good preparation for birth should build in an element of self-reliance, or foster reliance on a 'labour coach', a partner who has practised self-help methods with the woman and intends to be present during labour and delivery. Methods which rely heavily on the teacher's presence (for example, to provide a soothing commentary) are of limited value when the teacher is unlikely to be at the birth.

A teacher's methods may or may not be adapted to take account of her likely or certain absence from the scene of the action. They certainly do seem to be affected by her structural position in relation to the hospital.[15] Thus the midwives teaching in a hospital setting were seen to minimise patient choice; the physiotherapists, whether working in hospital or as voluntary childbirth teachers, encouraged women to use their initiative and the choices available to them. The physiotherapist working for the National Childbirth Trust outlined a wider range of choice than the hospital physiotherapist. The health visitor's teaching was affected by her limited information about the hospital, and instead of encouraging women to take an independent line, she tended to suggest that 'they' would look after the women she taught, so there was no need to worry. The community midwife, however, somewhat undermined this impression by her criticism of the administration of pain relief in hospital. This summary suggests that, while teaching will vary as a result of the relationship of teacher and hospital, it does not always vary in the same way. Those who work in the community may teach their group to trust the hospital staff, to fear them, or to assert themselves against the institutional tendency to standardise. Those who work in hospital may teach their group to conform to the system, or teach them how to use it to their advantage. Providing teachers have the knowledge, they can use their situation to suit their own aims.

They can also take into account the attitudes of the women they teach, providing they have established what these are. Encouraging women to use their initiative and exercise choice where this is possible may have different results for the socially competent woman supported by her husband, compared to the insecure, frightened, or aggressive unmarried mother. Similarly, general information on pain relief, for example, may be interpreted and used differently by a woman who fears excruciating pain and by one who fears oblivion at the birth. It is therefore helpful for staff to explore women's attitudes to hospital, labour and birth before offering teaching which may feed fears, rather than allay them. However, this explanation may itself be affected by their relationship with the hospital, in that women may be less willing to reveal fears of hospital practice, or medical interference, to staff who appear to them to be identified with the hospital itself. Where the class is held in the hospital and taught by staff in uniform, women may worry that revealing their fears will lead to ridicule, or being labelled an 'awkward' patient before they even try to assert themselves.

Possible Solutions to Structural Problems

It may too readily be assumed that to handle this difficulty all that a teacher needs is sensitivity, or a pleasant personality. While undoubtedly personal sensitivity to half-expressed fears will assist a teacher in assessing the expectations of the people in her group and teaching accordingly, this is a technical issue as well. If part of the problem in persuading people to express their fears is structural, in that some NHS teachers appear to be part of the system, then solutions which involve a structural component may be appropriate. The teacher could set up ways of detaching the information she wants about the range of views in the group, from the particular individuals who give it. There are several devices for doing this; the written, unsigned question to the teacher is perhaps the most obvious, though it is a method unlikely to be suited to small group work. Another possibility is the use of questions from the teacher to the group which do not demand a personal commitment to a belief, or fear, from the person who answers it; for example, 'Some people tell you a lot of odd things when you're pregnant, and they can worry you even if you don't really believe them — have you heard anything about induction, already?' A third way is to avoid individuals even having to express a fear in this remote way, and to divide the group into twos or threes to sort out lists of fears and worries which they, or pregnant women in general, might have. The teacher can then ask these smaller groups to raise these worries to be dealt with in the bigger group, so that all can benefit from the correction of misinformation. In the process, the teacher should find out a lot about what her group is worried about, and can slant her teaching to take account of these fears.

The second and third of these solutions depend on the teacher's ability to frame questions that will yield useful information. Claire Metcalf, working on research intended to establish women's expectations of postnatal care,[16] had the same problem, though beginning from a different standpoint. She found that general questions like 'What do you expect it to be like in hospital?' produced answers approximating to 'I don't know.' In a group, the effect is likely to be an embarrassing silence. Questioning needs to be more specific than this; she found, for example, that women did have expectations about whether staff would 'be too busy to deal with any problems or worries', would 'come round and ask if I am having any problems' and about whether they would be looked after by one or two nurses, or a lot of different staff, but they needed to be asked about these particular points. Using con-

trasting statements was effective in her research, and they are also useful in teaching — thus in group teaching on labour, such a question
might be: 'Do you expect the staff will be able to come round and ask
if you have any problems, or do you think they'll be too busy?' This
could usefully be followed up by the teacher's explanation of staff
allocation on the labour ward, the system for calling staff in emergency,
the extent to which patients are likely to be left alone, and other problems which may emerge as a result of the original question.

So far the assumption has been that the structural problems affecting teaching are concentrated in hospitals. Unfortunately for those who
work in the community, this is not the case. Where women go to a
community class, but will be delivered in hospital, they may well
wonder how much their teacher knows about the hospital — and sometimes doubts may even be justified.[17] Again, structural solutions need
to be sought for structural problems. One solution lies in more contact
by community staff with the hospital, organised either by individual
initiative or through in-service training. Another is the arrangement of
group reunions after the babies have arrived, so that the group can
exchange experiences and the teacher can learn by listening; some
community staff in the NHS use this system. The National Childbirth
Trust do this as well, and also ask women to write detailed reports on
their labours. A third lies in using the experience of women in the
group to provide an explicit bridge between hospital and community.
This is a possibility even with a group of women who are all expecting
their first baby; if they intend to give birth in hospital they are all
likely to have attended at least the hospital booking clinic, and may
have started to form expectations of hospital care based on this. Since
hospital clinics are frequently criticised as being rushed and imperso-
nal,[18] these expectations may be very worrying. If the teacher knows
that the labour ward and postnatal wards provide a more personal care,
she could correct this misunderstanding once it has been expressed and
supply supporting detail on staff allocation patterns, shifts, etc.

Preparation for childbirth has moved far since the days of Grantly
Dick Read. Technically it is more sophisticated, and therefore more
complicated to teach. But the teacher's responsibility does not end with
the understanding of the best time to use diaphragmatic breathing. If
she is to help each woman in her class to make the best use of these
techniques, she must attend both to the varied expectations of labour
with which women begin, and to the characteristics of two different
settings — that in which she herself teaches, and that in which the
women will give birth. Because much antenatal teaching is provided

in the NHS, finding out about expectations may demand more than goodwill; because many antenatal teachers do not also work on the labour ward, the attention to setting demands more than theoretical knowledge or previous experience. Antenatal teachers need to plan ways of making it easier for women to express their expectations and fears about labour, and ways in which they themselves can know enough about hospital practice to give detailed reassurance on specific points. Without such planning, preparation for childbirth risks becoming exercises in a vacuum, with little relationship either to the fears of the women who rely on them, or to the reality of the labours in which they are to be used.

Notes

1. Ann Oakley, 'The Baby Blues', *New Society* (5 April 1979), p. 11.
2. For methodological references, see Chapter 2, note 11.
3. See Chapter 2 for background on the National Childbirth Trust.
4. Patricia Hassid, *Textbook for Childbirth Educators* (Harper & Row, Hagerstown, Maryland, 1978), provides a detailed description of the various methods of physical preparation.
5. This comment was made during a tape-recorded interview which formed part of the study reported in Elizabeth R. Perkins, 'Having a Baby: An Educational Experience?', Occasional Paper 6 (Leverhulme Health Education Project, University of Nottingham, 1978); and in Elizabeth R. Perkins, 'Antenatal Care and Postnatal Nursing: Aspects of the Role of the Midwife in Health Education' in D.C. Anderson (ed.), *Health Education in Practice* (Croom Helm, London, 1979).
6. Herbert Benson with Miriam Z. Klipper, *The Relaxation Response* (Collins, London, 1976).
7. According to her managers.
8. Midwives require a doctor's consent, normally obtained in the last weeks of pregnancy, before administering any form of inhalation analgesia to patients.
9. As described in Chapter 2.
10. 'Many unpleasant experiences wrongly attributed to labour are caused by even small doses of pethidine in women not accustomed to hard drugs', K.O. Driscoll, J.M. Strange and M. Minogue, 'Active Management of Labour', *British Medical Journal*, vol. 3 (1977), pp. 135-7.
11. Michael Rosen, 'Pain and its Relief' in Tim Chard and Martin Richards (eds.), *Benefits and Hazards of the New Obstetrics: Clinics in Developmental Medicine*, no. 64 (Heinemann in association with Spastics International Medical Publications, London, 1977), supports this statement: 'In a number of trials it has been shown that 60 per cent or more of patients are completely satisfied, and 10 to 30 per cent reasonably satisfied with the method. Those who are not satisfied usually have a partial or failed block.'
12. Plain water is provided to avoid problems with glucose in the stomach, in case a general anaesthetic is required.
13. A.C. Breese, 'Antenatal Classes and Preparation for Pregnancy, Birth and Motherhood', unpublished MMedSci dissertation, University of Nottingham, 1976, states that 68.7 per cent of the sample of 150 women said they feared still-

birth or deformity during their pregnancies. Only 34.96 per cent sought help with this worry, and 63.4 per cent remained worried whether or not they had asked for help.

14. Grantly Dick Read, *Natural Childbirth* (Heinemann, London, 1933).

15. A similar argument, based on a different division of labour by professional staff, is developed in Jean Comaroff, 'Conflicting Paradigms of Pregnancy: Managing Ambiguity in Antenatal Encounters' in Alan Davies and Gordon Horobin (eds.), *Medical Encounters: The Experience of Illness and Treatment* (Croom Helm, London, 1977).

16. Claire Metcalf, personal communication (1979) based on unpublished research.

17. As the earlier details of the health visitor's ignorance of current hospital practice shows; health visitors' contact with hospital staff was found to be limited in a study described in Elizabeth R. Perkins, 'Antenatal Classes in Nottinghamshire: The Pattern of Official Provision', Occasional Paper 9 (Leverhulme Health Education Project, University of Nottingham, 1978).

18. For example, in Comaroff, 'Conflicting Paradigms of Pregnancy'; Perkins, 'Having a Baby: An Educational Experience?' and 'Antenatal Care and Postnatal Nursing: Aspects of the Role of the Midwife in Health Education'; and Hilary Graham, *The First Months of Motherhood*, vol. 4 Medical Care (University of York, 1979).

4 CLINIC BOOKLETS: HELP OR HINDRANCE IN PATIENT EDUCATION?

Elizabeth R. Perkins and Nicholas J. Spencer

Booklets and Their Uses

Parent education by books and booklets is by no means a new idea,[1] but there has recently been increased interest, at least from professionals, in this means of health education. This is shown by the publication of increasing numbers of child care leaflets and baby books,[2] by the development of non-academic short courses for parents by the Open University[3] and by various experiments in adapting the course material for a wider audience.[4] The attention given to parent education in the Court Report on the Child Health Services[5] may well have contributed to professional enthusiasm for the production and the distribution of literature on child care. The increase in volume has not, however, been accompanied by much public critical debate about the content and educational efficiency of the material available. In the belief that such a debate would contribute to an improvement in the quality of the literature,[6] this chapter sets out to examine one particular type of material, booklets distributed free through health service clinics. These booklets are an important source of advice to parents. Hilary Graham found that 99 per cent of her sample of 200 mothers in York were given the *You and Your Baby* booklets during their pregnancy, and that 38 per cent read in addition other literature on childbirth and child care. One month after the birth, 43 per cent of mothers reported reading child care literature since the baby's arrival, though 'those that did, tended to do so only in times of emergency'. By five months 67 per cent reported reading child care literature.[7]

These figures gain in significance when they are set against the possibilities for direct teaching by professional staff. Only about 45 per cent of expectant parents attend antenatal classes.[8] Antenatal clinics appear to be difficult places in which to teach effectively, judging by the studies which document some women's dissatisfaction with the information they receive.[9] After the birth, community midwives visit for a comparatively short time, and health visitors are usually unable to make very frequent home visits; the child health clinic is available as a source of professional advice, but some parents make little or no use of it.[10] Booklets therefore have advantages, both in the wide distribution possible through hospital or home visits just after birth, and in their availability as reference material when professionals are not present. They may also be used as handouts to reinforce advice already given by professional staff.

Since booklets could be given to parents at antenatal clinics, antenatal classes, in hospital, during home visits, and at child health clinics, the pattern of reception of these booklets is likely to be complicated, even when only initiatives by professionals are considered. In addition, many clinics set up literature displays where parents can help themselves. Here the attractiveness and readability of the booklets will presumably directly affect parental choice, not just later parental use of the literature. The choice of literature examined in this chapter has been governed by a simpler principle, that of one Area Health Authority's Health Education Unit's distribution pattern for 1978 (see Table 4.1). All references are to editions available in 1978. This is the main source of supply used by hospitals, health visitors and schools, and the figures can thus be used as a rough guide to the most popular pamphlets at that date.

Table 4.1: Distribution Pattern of Booklets and Leaflets, in One Area Health Authority, 1978

Breast Feeding	15,000
You and Your Baby, Parts I and II (booklets)	6,000 each
Protect Your Baby	6,000
Now You're a Family	6,000
Bottle Feeding? Let's Do It Right!	6,000
New Baby (booklet)	6,000
New Baby's First Three Years (booklet)	6,000
Weaning	5,000
You Know More Than You Think You Do	4,000
Bed Wetting	4,000
Care of Young Feet	4,000
Measles is Misery	4,000
Keep Baby Warm	4,000
Hello Baby!	4,000
You and Your Toothbrush	3,000
Now I am One Year Old	2,000
Your Children Need You	2,000
Can't Talk Yet?	2,000
Toys and Playthings: What Kind . . . At What Age?	2,000
Baby's Gone Metric	2,000
Scabies	2,000
The Overweight Child	2,000
Rubella	2,000
Total deliveries 1978	109,000

What this table cannot show is the reason for this popularity. It is possible, for example, that the wide distribution of *Breast Feeding* and of *Protect Your Baby*, which deals with immunisation, reflects the wish of professional staff to promote these activities. The booklets dealing with general problems of child rearing, such as the Health Visitors' Association's *New Baby* and *New Baby's First Three Years*, and the British Medical Association's *You and Your Baby*, Parts I and II, may reflect a pattern of distributing these to all expectant mothers attending particular classes or clinics. Further, staff will be likely to display and distribute what is available and free of cost, whether or not it is ideally suited to the purposes they have in mind. It would therefore be unsafe to use this table as an indicator either of parental choice or of the preferences of field staff. The figures are included as a quantitative backdrop to the essentially qualitative examination of the material which follows.

Information and Advice

Readers of pamphlets may expect both information about a problem and advice concerning it. These two functions of a pamphlet are distinct; it would be, for example, possible to write a pamphlet containing only information and leave parents to make up their own minds on the basis of this information, though the selection of information and its presentation would be likely to affect the decision made. Alternatively, pamphlets may provide advice without stating the reasons behind it. It is, therefore, interesting to see how this selection of pamphlets handles the interaction of information and advice.

One of the problems presented to the pamphlet writer is the nature of the research evidence available. Some is epidemiological only; sickness X often occurs in association with characteristic Y (e.g. weight at a particular age). Other evidence, of varying degrees of firmness, suggests that practice A causes, or contributes to, sickness X. Giving advice on the basis of these different types of evidence is not a simple matter. Some of the authors of these pamphlets have solved the problem by ignoring it. Instead of attempting to indicate the nature of the evidence on which their advice is based, they state that practice A is bad for babies — or even that characteristic Y is bad for babies.

The complicated subject of feeding advice illustrates this problem well. Bottle feeding carries with it certain dangers, the mechanism of which is understood and well established. Unsterile equipment means that the baby is vulnerable to infection; 'prop feeding' can result in a baby choking; excess milk powder risks dehydration during illness. None of these risks are explained in *Bottle feeding: Let's Do It Right*; instead mothers are given instructions:

> Don't ever leave him alone to feed by propping his bottle up in his cot or pram. It is vital that you maintain a warm physical contact while he is taking his bottle.

> The amount of milk powder and water has been carefully worked out so don't be tempted to make it stronger or weaker, or to add salt or sugar just because it seems tasteless to you.

This is good advice, but it invites obedience, not understanding.

The right time for introduction of solid foods is a more complex issue, but it is handled in the same basic way. *Weaning* states unequivocally:

> Whether baby is breast fed or bottle fed, milk is the only necessary food until the baby is four or even six months old. Don't listen to old wives' tales about starting solids any earlier. Rusks or other cereals given earlier won't make baby any healthier — and they may make him too fat.

The advice not to start solids before four months is based on three arguments. Early cereals may increase the likelihood of the baby developing coeliac disease, involving an inability to digest normal flour;[11] giving solids not accompanied by extra liquid increases the risk of dehydration if the baby is ill;[12] solids may make the baby fat. Only the third possibility is mentioned in *Weaning* in connection with the timing of the introduction of solid foods. However, kidney damage is given as a reason for not adding salt to food, and overweight babies and future tooth decay (as a result of an acquired taste for sugar) as a reason for not adding sugar.

This leaflet assumes that it is accepted that babies should not be 'overweight' or 'too fat'. The choice of words certainly makes it difficult for anyone to argue in favour of being 'too fat'. This disapproval of overweight babies is based on two principles not articulated in the pamphlets, that a fat baby is not a fit baby, and that fat babies make fat adults. The first is based on evidence suggesting that heavier children are more prone to infection.[13] The second, based on research suggesting that fat cells laid down in childhood persist into adulthood, is more problematic. Recent studies have severely dented this theory by demonstrating on long-term follow-up studies that only 20 per cent of children who are overweight at six months remain overweight at four years.[14]

The prescriptive tone of the extract from *Weaning* is therefore not fully justified by recent research findings. Even if it was, the failure to explain why the early introduction of solid foods is so reprehensible does not help a mother faced with an unsatisfied baby of about three months old. She knows what the baby's crying is doing to her and the baby. She is not told what damage she will be doing if she adds a rusk to his bottle. She therefore has no evidence on which she can balance the risks of making her baby a little heavier against those of his persistent crying. Nor is she offered alternative ways of handling the problem, except for the suggestion that the baby is thirsty and should be given boiled water or fruit juice. Yet since the introduction of solid foods appears to be undertaken mainly as a solution to specific feeding difficulties,[15] clear explanation of what the risks are, and alternative suggestions for dealing with the problem, would seem to be essential if mothers are to be expected to take the advice which the pamphlet gives.

The timing of the introduction of solid foods is one example of recent professional controversy. The fact that professionals can, and frequently do, give different advice is not mentioned in the booklets, and the impression is given of uniformity of professional opinion. However, the problems which parents find with conflicting advice are well documented by a number of studies,[16] and indeed, it is difficult to see how this can be avoided on some issues, where the evidence is by no means unequivocal. New research, and professional disagreement about good practice, clearly present a challenge to the writers of child care literature, as well as a problem to the parents for whom they write. It does not, however, help mothers, or improve the credibility of the literature, to pretend that these problems do not exist. Fewer forthright statements of 'good practice', and more explanations of why practice A is at present thought to be more beneficial than practice B, would provide a framework within which different types of advice could be incorporated, and would help parents to make decisions with a better understanding of the balance of risks. Such an approach would also reduce the risks to the producers of literature. Consider, for example, two extracts from *You and Your Baby*. In Part II the following statement on breast feeding occurs in the 1978 edition:

For the first two or three days there is generally very little milk. Just
a flow of thin colostrum. Therefore there is little point in putting
baby to the breast for more than just a few brief moments. But this
is well worthwhile because it allows colostrum to be removed and
gives both mother and baby some practice in the more serious business of feeding that follows.

Contrast this with the following:

When the baby is born, many midwives allow him to suckle for a
few seconds shortly after birth. This also helps the womb to return
to its normal size more quickly. The baby should be put to the
breast again — for about half a minute on each side — in about four
hours, and again about four hours later for a minute each side. This
process is continued until, at the end of twenty four hours, the baby
is having quite a good feed.

Two completely different approaches appear in sister publications.
The first would now be regarded as frankly inaccurate by scientists who
have studied colostrum[17] and it is a good example of poor editing as
well as of the rapidity with which so-called scientific facts change. The
1979 edition omits this first passage. The second is closer to the
presently accepted approach, but many paediatricians would argue with
aspects of it, particularly the insistence on a four hourly feeding
regime.[18]

Advice Without Evidence

The advice we have examined so far is based on evidence, some strong,
some weak and some scientifically obsolete. These pamphlets also give
advice not based on evidence. Some is based on experience of similar
situations — sample menus as in *Weaning*, suggestions for diets and
sandwich lunches as in *The Overweight Child*, or suitable toys as in
Toys and Playthings. Advice of this kind is on a level with advice from
experienced mothers who have faced the same situation, and say 'I
found this worked well'. *The Overweight Child* makes this clear in its
subheading 'Some helpful tips'. In *Weaning*, however, the sample
menus are headed 'Starting solids', and breast or bottle feeds disappear
between five and seven months. There is, however, no explanation or
justification for this arbitrary timing. The end of breast feeding is a

matter of personal preference, not of prescription.

A fourth type of advice is apparently based neither on evidence nor on practical experience, but on cultural patterns. *The Overweight Child* states:

> Meal times can be just as important for nourishing family life as well as our bodies. A child should eat his meals sitting down with at least one other person, either you, a brother or sister. Try and set aside a regular number of days or times when meals can be family occasions.

Your Children Need You states that children need 'a regular bedtime to help them establish good sleeping habits', but it is not clear what 'good' means here. There are several arguments in favour of family meals and regular bedtimes: the promotion of table manners; parental peace in the evenings; the benefits of a particular routine for the child. The pamphlets, however, give no clue to their reasoning. Both examples suggest that what is really being said is that many people (including the author) think family meals and regular bedtimes for children are part of normal family life.

A further subdivision of this type of advice seems to be based on the norms of a very small subcultural group indeed, expanded to become 'most women think', as in *You and Your Baby*, Part I:

> Most women think it is nature's design for the baby to be suckled at the breast for the first two or three weeks. Whether they feel it is natural or even fashionable to go on feeding their babies is another matter.

It is difficult to see what basis the writer can have for this statement. To begin with, it is contradictory; either breast feeding is felt to be 'natural' or it is not. Why should women be expected to feel that it is unnatural after two weeks? They may well decide that it is inconvenient, or inefficient, at this stage, but this is another matter. The large scale study of infant feeding carried out in 1975 showed that most mothers who stopped breast feeding in the first six weeks used physical factors as the main reason for doing so, rather than personal and social factors. Further, the research showed a clearly defined factor of 'distaste for breast feeding', which is far stronger, as one might expect, among mothers who bottle fed completely than it is among mothers who breast fed completely, or among those who stopped breast feeding in the first six weeks. Neither type of evidence provides support for the idea that

an appreciable number of women find breast feeding natural for a
period of two weeks.[19]

'Most women think' statements may, perhaps, represent the views
of the author's women friends. This interpretation is strengthened by
the presence of paragraphs of advice like the following, from *You and
Your Baby*, Part II, where the 'explanatory' start is missing:

> Have your hair done within one or two weeks of delivery, and get
> yourself a new dress now that you are much slimmer. You should
> certainly get out with your husband and enjoy yourself from time to
> time . . . In conclusion you will rightly expect your husband to be
> loving towards you and admire your recent achievement! But
> remember that he has been deprived of your company (and sex) for
> a long time and see to it that the new member of the family does not
> mean that he has less of your time and love.

The effect of this advice on the single girl, on the couple for whom the
pregnancy was a financial disaster, and who could, therefore, not
afford hairdresser's prices, new clothes, and babysitters, or on the
woman whose marriage is breaking up, has only to be imagined to be
deplored. Furthermore, the imperative tone is again being applied in
matters which are patently nothing to do with medical authority. A
hairdresser's shop might be the last place a woman would want to go,
even if she was able to arrange for an afternoon out without the baby.
It is a matter of choice, and indeed, this could be what a mother needs
most from a free afternoon. 'Most women think' statements are totally
uneducational; those based on larger subcultural groups may be useful
to those who share the norms of the writer. Both cases are products of
a failure on the part of the authors to think clearly about the basis for
the advice they give, and to make this basis clear in their writing.

Confusing Information

On occasion, a writer may appear to be so heavily committed to giving
advice rather than information that when advice is inappropriate he
seems incapable of giving comprehensible explanations.

You and Your Baby, Part I, strongly advises mothers to attend for
antenatal care, using subheadings like 'Time to see your doctor'. It then
refers to the procedures which will be carried out in the antenatal
clinics. Here information is essential. However, when one examines

some of the 'explanations' offered, for example on Rhesus incompatibility, information is singularly hard to find:

> It also shows whether your blood does or does not contain what we call Rhesus factor. If your blood does contain this factor, then your blood is Rhesus-positive. If it does not, then your blood is Rhesus-negative. If your child's blood is Rhesus-positive and your own is Rhesus-negative, steps can now be taken to remedy the matter during your antenatal care.

Clearly women could ask for explanations of this problem, but the booklets are presumably written to fill the education gap. Rhesus factor could be anything from a hormone to a cosmetic in competition with Max Factor for all this booklet explains. Far worse is the nonsense about steps being taken in antenatal care to remedy Rhesus incompatibility. The problem of Rhesus incompatibility is a genuine worry for many expectant mothers, although there is no direct threat to the life of the foetus in the first pregnancy. However, if a Rhesus-negative mother has a first Rhesus-positive child and a subsequent foetus is also Rhesus-positive, there is a risk to this child from maternal antibodies developed during the earlier pregnancy. The situation is therefore monitored, *not* remedied, in antenatal care during *each* pregnancy, by checking on the level of maternal antibodies. An injection is given soon after delivery to those mothers with significant antibody levels, and this should prevent problems in the next pregnancy. Only in rare, severe cases of established Rhesus disease would action be taken during antenatal care, when intra-uterine exchange transfusions − difficult, last resort procedures − can be carried out in a few expert centres.

The above example is a particularly glaring example of the withholding of information. The 1979 edition does avoid telling mothers that Rhesus incompatibility can be remedied in antenatal care, but it still does not explain what Rhesus factor is.

Advice and its Uses

These booklets contain a mixture of advice based on good evidence, advice based on equivocal evidence, helpful hints and statements of cultural or subcultural norms. Reasons for the advice proffered are frequently absent. Parents have thus no means of discriminating between instructions based on good evidence and those based on sub-

cultural norms which they do not share, and may throw out the baby
with the subcultural bathwater. It is, however, possible to avoid the pit-
falls of muddling different types of advice; the pamphlet *Bed Wetting* is
a good illustration of this. It recognises that most parents find this
problem upsetting and explains why bed wetting occurs, how it can be
tackled, details the parents' and the doctor's part in its management,
and also gives information on the scope of the problem in different age
groups. Similarly, *Protect Your Baby* and *Rubella* provide facts about
the disease against which immunisation is offered, how to arrange
immunisation, side effects and possible contra-indications to be reported to the doctor before immunisation is given. The vexed question of
the extent of the risk of whooping cough vaccination, however, is not
discussed in *Protect Your Baby*; parents are referred to their doctor or
health visitor. Since the whole problem is that the medical profession
has disagreed violently and publicly on the risks involved, this does not
seem very helpful. A leaflet detailing the arguments would be easier
to use as an aid to decision-making by parents than a chat with a health
professional who may be busy, who may not have the information
readily available, and who may not believe that the parents should be
provided with information anyway.

The Relationship with the Health Services

The services are portrayed as faultless, friendly, instantly available and
easily approachable. Antenatal clinics, child health clinics, midwives,
health visitors and general practitioners are all given the same image of
excellence. It is almost as if the booklet writers have been dreaming of
a perfect health service and, on waking, have immediately committed
their dreams to paper. Presenting this untarnished, irreproachable image
has at least two disadvantages. First, most parents are quite aware that
problems do exist with the services and the bland implication that the
relationship between provider and consumer is always an easy one just
does not ring true. Secondly, by implying that the official services are
the natural, or even the only, advice sources, the booklets could effectively diminish parental regard for the sources they find easiest to use,
the experience of mother, neighbour or friend, without providing any
help for parents who are nervous of using the professional services.

Some examples will serve to illustrate these general points. The
BMA publication, *You and Your Baby*, Part I, manages to convey the
idea of perfect services at the same time as being embarrassingly patron-

ising. It states:

> You decide when to see your doctor and let him confirm the fact
> of your pregnancy. From then onwards you are going to have to
> answer a lot of questions and be the subject of a lot of examinations.
> Never worry your head about any of these. They are necessary, they
> are in the interests of your baby and yourself, and none of them will
> ever hurt you.

As one would expect from a BMA publication, *You and Your Baby*,
Part I, is determined to paint a rosy picture of the general practitioner:
'If you have any questions to ask or any special worries, don't hesitate
to go and see your family doctor. I am sure he will see that your questions are fully answered.' The author may be sure that the family
doctor will fully answer all questions, but it is doubtful whether a significant minority of mothers are also as sure, judging by their accounts of
the antenatal period reported in a small number of studies.[20] To
parents of small children who have struggled with receptionists for the
privilege of even *seeing* the doctor such assertions must have a rather
hollow ring.

The implication that the natural advice sources are the official
services is clear in the above quotations. In *You Know More Than You
Think You Do*, a generally excellent booklet written by Claire Rayner,
non-professional advice sources are roundly condemned and professional sources uncritically supported. When trying to persuade mothers
to have their children immunised, Claire Rayner writes:

> Listen to the advice your doctor or health visitor gives on this matter
> — *never* to the uninformed gossip of neighbours or others who might
> try to put you off accepting immunisations for your child. They are
> necessary for his health. So there is another basic: USE ALL THE
> AVAILABLE EXPERT ADVICE OFFERED AT YOUR CLINIC:
> it's the best there is . . . (emphasis and capitals as in the original.)

The Health Visitors' Association booklet *New Baby* goes further
than most in recognising that problems with services do exist. However,
instead of dealing fully with these problems, and suggesting ways for
parents to overcome them, they tend to put the onus entirely on the
parent as in the following extract:

> So if you are anxious, concerned, or merely curious about what is

happening to you during pregnancy, speak to those who are looking after you. Crowded surgeries and heavily booked antenatal clinics aren't always the easiest places in which to discuss a problem. You will find some more ready than others to answer your questions. It's up to you to find the answers affecting your own pregnancy from the people who are caring for you.

Because no attempt is made actively to advise parents on how to make use of the services, booklets such as *New Baby* can only suggest what would be beneficial for parents without telling them how to go about getting it. When discussing fathers attending the birth the booklet says:

> Some hospitals are happy to have fathers present at the confinement. Others are not at all keen. Check this point in good time if it matters a lot to both of you. It is possible for the closest family bond to develop right from the start if couples take on parenthood together.

The ideal situation is stated, the problems are recognised, but no attempt is made to help parents to overcome the problems and achieve the ideal.

If it is accepted that the presentation of the health services in these booklets is somewhat unrealistic, it is reasonable to go on to consider how else they could be portrayed and what advice parents could be given about using them. Writers may fear to present an unnecessarily critical picture of the services. However, those parents with access to excellent services would have no need of encouragement from booklets to make use of them, and those with unsatisfactory services would feel that the booklets more accurately reflected their circumstances. While it may not be easy either to write fairly and realistically about the services or to suggest ways of making use of them, attempts have already been made to tackle this problem in the Open University course material *The First Years of Life*. The topic 'Questions at your antenatal clinic' in Book 2 gives women a preview of the questions asked, and encourages them to formulate their own questions. In addition, it gives a list of people the woman is likely to meet in the clinic, and a brief outline of their functions, in order that she can decide who to ask about what. 'Going to your baby clinic' in Book 4 accepts that mothers may perceive disadvantages as well as advantages in attending any particular clinic, and offers a check list to help mothers make their own decisions about individual local clinics. Unfortunately the course material is not currently available for free distribution and some of the existing booklets would have to change their approach radically to incorporate information of this sort.

Decision-making

Providing information implies a hope that parents will use it. The simultaneous provision of advice shows the way in which the author hopes parents will use it. The limited information on whooping cough vaccine in *Protect Your Baby*, and the referral to doctor or health visitor, is symptomatic of a general trend in these pamphlets. Rarely is a decision articulated clearly and left with the parents as their responsibility. In *Bottle Feeding: Let's Do It Right*, variations on the advice to consult midwife or health visitor appear nine times in six pages — it is tempting to wonder why the leaflet was written in the first place, if advice is so easy to come by in person and so difficult to convey in print. Only two of the pamphlets studied explicitly set out to help parents to take their own decisions: *Toys and Playthings: What Kind . . . At What Age?*, and *Breast Feeding*, a pamphlet produced by the National Association for Maternal and Child Welfare. *Breast Feeding*, indeed, begins with a choice — 'Three ways of feeding the baby'. It details arguments for breast and bottle feeding, considers the idea of combining both methods, and comments: 'There is no proof that any of the three ways of infant feeding is, for most mothers, a great deal better than any other.'

The conclusion to this section begins: 'It is for the mother to decide which way she wants to feed her baby.' It then goes on to provide detailed information on the production of breast milk, feeding routines, care of the breasts, what to do if the baby is still hungry, and vitamin supplements. In dealing with solid foods and weaning from the breast the authors sensibly begin 'The mother will decide how long she wants to breast feed'. This leaflet gives plenty of information and places the decisions firmly where they belong — with the mother.

The Health Education Council's leaflet on children's toys combines information on children's play development at each stage, with a list 'Suitable toys include: . . .' This leaflet explicitly classifies many of its ideas as suggestions both at the beginning, 'The following suggestions will help you to make the right choice', and later on, 'It is a good idea to have a new toy handy for special occasions, illness or disappointment'.

It also, however, includes some very directive advice. For three- to
four-year-olds, it comments:

> More than ever, your child will now enjoy playing with other chil-
> dren of his own age. You should make this possible and also en-
> courage opportunities for exploration and physical exercise, indoors
> and out.

This is, in itself, sensible advice. However, the way in which it is
phrased defines the normal range of behaviour of three-year-olds in such
a way as to exclude the very shy child — 'Your child *will now enjoy* . . .'
This extract goes on to direct parents in what they should do, rather
than leaving them to draw their own conclusions from their children's
enjoyment of the company of others. It does not explain in what
other ways such company will benefit their child; the rationale for the
use of the imperative would presumably be that other children's company will help in social development. Similarly, in the section 'How
many toys', it is stated:

> Many of your child's playthings, as we have seen, will be improvised
> from everyday objects. But he will need some toys from the toy-
> shop. There is no reason to give him a great number of them.

It is not made clear why a child 'needs' toys from the toyshop; the
quantity of such toys is surely a matter for parents to decide. At the
end of the pamphlet, 'A Final Word' lapses again into the habit of
instructing parents:

> Toys and playthings, as we have seen, are an essential part of
> growing up. But no aspect of a child's play is more important than
> the time he spends playing with mother and father. Make sure that
> you spend some time, during the day or evening, playing with the
> children.

Here we have the familiar pattern of instruction without explanation —
an incongruous end to a pamphlet which starts off as an aid to parent
decision-making.

Aids to Decision-making

Pregnant women and parents do not make decisions in a vacuum. They use the information they have, inadequate though this may be, together with their intuitive understanding of the problem with which they are faced.

Claire Rayner, in *You Know More Than You Think You Do*, states 'This booklet sets out to help you discover and use the knowledge you don't know you have'. The pamphlet provides background information on mothers and babies: their ways of communicating, their delight in cuddles, their reactions to feeding and feeding problems. Within this framework the writer encourages mothers to trust their own instincts and their babies' reactions. This approach involves both providing information and encouraging mothers to be honest about their own feelings.

In *Now You're a Family*, Claire Rayner gives a range of alternative feelings people might have, thus implicitly recognising the width of the range, and helping a woman to sort out which of these feelings she has. Other booklets tell women what they will, or should, feel. *You and Your Baby*, Part I, for example, exhorts women to: 'Remember that pregnancy should be regarded as a normal female function which should be enjoyable as well as memorable as you especially can make it become so.' A woman with bad morning sickness is thus told that first she should be enjoying pregnancy, and that secondly, it is her own fault if she is not enjoying it! A possibly more damaging example is found in the 1978 edition of *New Baby*: 'Although the routine may seem tough, you will feel reasonably confident about coping with the new baby, when you leave the hospital.' Panic on returning home with a new baby is by no means unusual; anyone turning to a booklet for help will hardly be comforted to be told that in fact she feels reasonably confident!

If mothers have knowledge about themselves and their new babies, which only needs to be recognised and thus made available to them, how much more do they have knowledge about their own bodies in pregnancy? While changes in pregnancy can be bewildering, it is possible to relate many of them either to a general slowing of bodily functions, or to physical or mental efforts to adjust to the pregnancy. If, as *You and Your Baby*, Part I, argues: 'Pregnancy is not an illness — more an unusual state of normality — even though it may seem a little strange at first', women should be encouraged to look for continuity with their pre-pregnant state, rather than to treat pregnancy as a new phenomenon where none of the old commonsense rules apply.

Intermittently, these booklets recognise the uses of continuity. *New Baby*, on exercise in pregnancy, states, 'Your own body will tell you how far to go'. It also refers to the 'natural brake' which pregnancy may apply to a woman's consumption of cigarettes, drugs and alcohol, so that she does not want excessive quantities, as well as explaining why smoking and drugs are harmful in pregnancy. On intercourse in the weeks immediately after delivery, it continues this approach, but without the supporting information which may be needed to give women confidence to do so: 'It is safe purely from the physical point of view to resume intercourse when both parties are ready.' Since it is not at all clear what 'ready' means here, whether the end of bleeding, or revival of interest, this is a singularly unhelpful statement.

If *New Baby* sometimes runs the risk of stressing trust in a woman's instincts at the expense of information, *You and Your Baby*, predictably, over-balances in the opposite direction. Its effect is complicated by the considerable variations in style among its contributors. Some sections credit a woman with commonsense. Others adopt the patronising attitude to a woman's own understanding of her body apparent in the first section on conception: 'No doctor could ever dispute the highly unscientific accuracy of most feminine intuition'. In spite of such unpromising phrases, 'Dos and don'ts in pregnancy' relates life in pregnancy firmly to life beforehand: the remarks on exercise, rest, and sex are good examples of this approach. The section on 'Keeping well — coping with minor problems', however, does not continue it. It starts with a clear statement of the problems minor ailments can cause:

> They tend to be worrying because the woman and her friends and relatives don't understand how and why they came about, don't understand their meaning, and consequently fear that their symptoms may mean that something has gone wrong.

While this section carries out its stated task of explaining why minor discomforts happen, it does not, in general, encourage women to relate their own problems to their own previous experience. Palpitations and breathlessness, for example, are stated to be of emotional origin; since these are common stress symptoms in or out of pregnancy, it might have been useful to point this out. Similarly, dizziness on getting up suddenly is not confined to pregnant women. The only attempt made in this section to encourage women to refer back to past experience is on vaginal discharge:

always increased in pregnancy . . . like the normal white discharge of the non-pregnant woman even though increased in amount. Other whitish or yellowish discharges are caused by minor infections of the skin of the vagina. They cause soreness or itching around the outside and should be reported to the doctor . . .

This is an excellent example of the way in which women can be helped to use their past experience to decide what is worth reporting to their doctor and what is not. The tendency to encourage a conceptual divorce between pre-pregnancy and pregnancy is likely to result in unnecessary anxiety for pregnant women, which they may or may not relieve by asking their doctors or midwives.

Thus, decision-making can be facilitated by material that recognises and builds on the knowledge and previous experience of those for whom the material is intended. Unfortunately many of the booklets fail to adopt this approach consistently and, by the same token, fail to recognise other sorts of experience, the problems and difficulties with which families have to cope.

The Family Setting

With a few notable exceptions, the booklets are written as if life takes place in a vacuum, without any of the conflicts, contradictions and difficulties of the real world. All babies seem to be born into happy families, and have well housed and financially solvent parents. Babies are always planned and are never conceived, let alone born, before their mothers are married. Single-parent families do not exist, and fathers are falling over themselves to carry out their paternal duties. The only apparent problem in this idyllic setting is that all the parents are simple-minded and so have to be told that their children need them (*Your Children Need You*) and that babies kept in bath water too long will get cold (*You and Your Baby*, Part II).

Though this caricature is undoubtedly a little cruel, there is ample evidence in the booklets of a failure by the authors to show that they appreciate the reality of life for many young families. Even the most 'responsible' middle-class parents would be hard pressed to identify with the perfect couples depicted in some of the booklets.

You and Your Baby, Part II, starts with the seemingly innocuous sentence: 'Now you and your husband and this tiny baby that you have been thinking about and waiting for all these months are a real family.'

However, the underlying implications are far from innocuous. It takes a husband to make 'a real family'; therefore single-parent families are excluded from being 'real' and the unmarried mother need read no further! At no time in this publication is any recognition given to the single-parent family and its particular difficulties.

The early pages of the HVA publication *New Baby* tend to fall into the same trap. There is constant reference to the importance of the husband, for example: 'A husband's help and encouragement can be a woman's biggest prop during her pregnancy and the birth.'

Not only may the single mother be excluded by implication; so may poor parents. Advertisements contribute to this effect in the BMA and HVA booklets. For example the Baby Boots advertisement on pages 6 and 7 of *New Baby* asks 'Just what does it take to be a good mum'. In other words, good mothering is judged by financial standing and the ability to buy Boots products. Other advertisements are peopled by attractive, beautifully dressed young couples photographed in their chic homes or standing near their expensive cars.

It could be argued that the effect of advertising, while possibly deplorable, is not the responsibility of the writers of these booklets. However, a similar standard of living is indicated in illustrations in literature produced by the Health Education Council. *Keep Baby Warm*, for example, has an informative text, but depicts on the back cover a bedroom which is apparently to be occupied only by the baby. The walls are painted in toning shades, with matching curtains, lampshade, and floor coverings. It is larger than the small single rooms found in many new houses. While the colouring is no doubt influenced by printing costs as well as designer's choice, the effect is certainly not one of second-hand furniture and a tight budget.

Ignoring the special problems of poor or single-parent families risks such parents deciding that the booklets are not relevant to any of their difficulties. Such a decision could be misguided, deriving from a confusion of standard of living and family composition with medical advice. The writers' presentation of advice in the context of the 'normal' family does, however, result in some material which really is unrealistic. Families in cramped accommodation, living with in-laws, or living in thin-walled rooms next to neighbours who complain every time the baby cries, are bound to take these realities into account in their daily decisions on feeding methods, child rearing practices, and frequency of intercourse. Yet breast feeding, for example, is presented in these pamphlets as *the* natural choice and praise is liberally showered on mothers choosing this method, with no reference to the embarrassment and distaste that some mothers would have to overcome — for example, a young insecure mother trying to breast feed her baby with mother and father-in-law, not to mention grandfather-in-law in the same house, or even in the same room. By ignoring such problems a valuable opportunity is missed to suggest possible solutions, or at least to provide these mothers with some encouragement by simply recognising that their difficulties exist.

Many families do not experience the kind of social privations mentioned above, but they almost without exception face conflicts and contradictions in their role as parents. These conflicts provide one of the main themes of Claire Rayner's two booklets — *You Know More Than You Think You Do* and *Now You're a Family*. It is the open and full discussion of the potential stresses of parenthood that makes these booklets most suitable for those mothers whose social difficulties leave them particularly vulnerable to conflicts and stresses. There is considerable evidence[21] linking high levels of maternal stress with illness both in the mother and her baby, and though the discussion of such stress in booklets cannot hope to alleviate the basic problems, it can help in giving mothers insight into their difficulties, and the knowledge that they are not alone in being so troubled. This is a far more realistic and sensible approach than to present a dream world of happy families served by an always excellent health service.

Conclusion

It is reasonable to assume that booklets on babies, aimed at parents, are intended to be educational literature, particularly when they are issued by such bodies as the Health *Education* Council. If education is concerned with providing information which the recipient can use to make his or her own decisions, a number of these booklets are only intermittently educational. First, the quality of the information offered is in some cases suspect. A small proportion is frankly inaccurate, as in the 1978 BMA booklet's statements on Rhesus incompatibility and colostrum. Far more common, however, is the tendency to provide advice without indicating the kind of information on which it is based, and to use as a basis for advice research which is not always unequivocally established, without making this clear, as in the material on solid foods. The failure to consider seriously the basis of the advice offered culminates in the idiocy of advising women to have their hair done with the same seriousness as advising them to sterilise baby feeding bottles.

If advice was not given without supporting reasons, this sort of error would be avoided. Secondly, making decisions is not a skill which is fostered by many of these booklets. Some try to pre-empt the decisions, for example by telling people which feeding method to use, or what toys to buy. This may be done directly, or by the use of vocabulary which indicates the shamefulness of the alternative choice. Others denigrate parental instinct and knowledge, urging them with monotonous regularity to ask the professionals. The unwillingness to leave decisions where they properly belong, with the parents, may leave an impression, in the minds of some parents, of officious impertinence, and in the minds of others, a simple, often unconscious, determination to take no notice of whatever advice is given. Yet a further group may accept medical authority without questioning its basis, and obey without understanding. Since child rearing is not a matter of carrying out simple instructions to order, this is not a good means of improving family life. Thirdly, in trying to write for all parents many of the authors have ignored the fact that all parents are different and live in different circumstances. The failure to give much, or in some cases any, consideration to the problems of single parents, teenagers living with in-laws, or couples in bad housing, lays a considerable burden on these parents to adapt advice suited to a well-housed couple in their twenties to their own difficult circumstances. This task of adaptation is not easy and it would not be at all surprising if these parents decided not to try. Furthermore, successful education depends on the learner's motivation. Literature which patronises, induces guilt or anxiety, or encourages feelings of social inferiority, is unlikely to enhance parents' willingness to learn. Some of these booklets use stylistic devices which could have this effect on parents.

At this point we must insert one caveat. We have argued that the booklets we examined *can* be read in particular ways, and that these readings are likely to discourage active learning, rather than to encourage it. This is, of course, not the same thing as proving that all parents *do* read the booklets in the same way, and, indeed, we have argued that the effect of literature on parents is likely to be related to the extent to which this literature appears to reflect their particular circumstances. Finding out how parents *do* read this literature requires a different sort of evidence, that collected from parents themselves; it is interesting that the recommendations of the First Months of Motherhood project at York, based on evidence from mothers, includes:

Specifically, we suggest that official information should also be more regularly up-dated to take account of changing ideas, practices, and that mothers' criticisms should be incorporated into all recent publications. Information about weaning and child development were two areas where mothers often found the observations old-fashioned.[22]

It seems, therefore, that our reading of this literature cannot be dismissed as idiosyncratic. Even if only a minority of parents shared our perspective on this literature, we consider that the risks of discouraging active learning are sufficient to make a review of these publications overdue. Clinic booklets should be an aid to parents, and to busy professionals, in their task as health educators; some of the range available in 1978 do not seem to us to deserve such a description.

While those who write clinic booklets consider their position, professionals will no doubt continue to find booklets useful in their daily work. What are the implications of our criticisms for them? We suggest two lines of action. Professionals who use booklets as an aid to themselves (in busy clinics) and their clients (as an ever-present help in time of trouble) should first read them. We find it difficult to believe that Chamberlain and Chave,[23] who describe *You and Your Baby* as a 'well written, authoritative and attractively presented magazine' can have read it recently; some of the material is no longer authoritative, and a more appropriate word might be 'authoritarian'. Having read them, they may still decide to use them — but as part of a teaching session, not as a substitute for one. *Bottle Feeding: Let's Do It Right*, for example, would be much less objectionable used as a check list for reference after a class, than it would be as a handout on how to bottle feed. Professionals have to work with the literature available, and in some circumstances almost any leaflet may be better than none. However, they would benefit from a wider choice of leaflets which really are educational tools, and a reduction in the number which are only pretending.

Notes

1. For example, L. Emmett Holt, *Care and Feeding of Infants* (D. Appleton & Co., New York and London, 1896).

2. For example, well established 'baby books': R.S. Illingworth and C. Illingworth, *Babies and Young Children*, 6th edn (Churchill Livingstone, Edinburgh, 1978); B. Spock, *Baby and Child Care* (Bodley Head, London, 1958). Recent additions: P. Leach, *Babyhood* (Pelican Books, London, 1974); P. Leach, *Baby and Child* (Michael Joseph, London, 1977); P. Fenwick and C. Fenwick, *The Baby Book for Fathers* (Angus & Robertson, Brighton, 1978).

3. *The First Years of Life* and *The Preschool Child* (1977).

4. For example, the production of short leaflets and the development with the Scottish Health Education Unit of *The Book of the Child*. For details, see Nick Farnes (ed.), *Community Education with the Open University*, provisional edn (Open University, Milton Keynes, May 1979).

5. Report of the Committee on Child Health Services, *Fit for the Future* (HMSO, London, 1976).

6. The evaluation schemes for the Open University materials were designed with this aim, among others, in mind.

7. Hilary Graham, *The First Months of Motherhood* (University of York, 1979).

8. The figure of 45 per cent is compounded from the results of various studies: E.R. Perkins, 'Attendance at Antenatal Classes: A District Study', Occasional Paper 13 (Leverhulme Health Education Project, University of Nottingham, 1979); G. Chamberlain, 'Antenatal Education', *Midwife, Health Visitor and Community Nurse*, vol. 11 (September 1975), p. 289; D.A. Mandelstam, 'The Value of Antenatal Preparation – A Statistical Survey', *Midwife and Health Visitor*, vol. 7 (June 1971), p. 217; N.J. Spencer, 'The Identification and Management of Illness by Parents of Young Children', unpublished MPhil thesis, University of Nottingham, presented 1980. B.M. Hibbard *et al.*, in 'The Effectiveness of Antenatal Education', *Health Education Journal*, vol. 38, no. 2 (1979), pp. 39-46, classified only 28 per cent of their sample primigravidae as attenders, but their definition of attendance required women to go to at least 75 per cent of mothercraft classes; thus the figures are not comparable.

9. For example, Graham, *The First Months of Motherhood*; Elizabeth R. Perkins, 'Antenatal Care and Postnatal Nursing: Aspects of the Role of the Midwife in Health Education' in D.C. Anderson (ed.), *Health Education in Practice* (Croom Helm, London, 1979); Spencer, 'The Identification and Management of Illness by Parents of Young Children'; Elizabeth R. Perkins, 'Having a Baby: An Educational Experience?', Occasional Paper 6 (Leverhulme Health Education Project, University of Nottingham, 1978).

10. Report of the Committee on Child Health Services, *Fit for the Future*; Graham, *The First Months of Motherhood*.

11. G.C. Amerl, J.H. Hutchinson and R.A. Shanks, Personal Communication to the Working Party of the Panel on Child Nutrition, Committee on Medical Aspects of Food Policy, reported in DHSS, *Present Day Practice in Infant Feeding*, Report on Health and Social Subjects, no. 9 (HMSO, London, 1974).

12. D.P. Davies, 'Osmolality Homeostasis and Renal Function in Infancy', *Postgraduate Medical Journal*, vol. 51 supplement 3 (1975), pp. 25-30; L.S. Taitz and H.D. Byers, 'High Coloria/osmolen Feeding and Hypertonic Dehydration', *Archives of Disease in Childhood*, vol. 47 (1972), p. 257.

13. B. Hutchinson-Smith, 'The Relationship Between the Weight of an Infant and Lower Respiratory Infection', *Medical Officer*, vol. 123 (1970), pp. 257-62.

14. E.M.E. Poskitt and T.J. Cole, 'Nature, Nurture and Childhood Overweight', *British Medical Journal*, vol. 1 (1978), pp. 603-5.

15. Graham, *The First Months of Motherhood*; Jean Martin, *Infant Feeding 1975: Attitudes and Practice in England and Wales* (HMSO, London, 1978).

16. Ann Cartwright, *Human Relations and Hospital Care* (Routledge & Kegan Paul, London, 1964); Hazel Houghton, 'Problems of Hospital Communication' in Gordon McLachlan (ed.), *Problems and Progress in Medical Care: Essays on Current Research*, 3rd series (Oxford University Press, London, 1968); Gaynor D. MacLean, 'An Appraisal of the Concepts of Infant Feeding and their Application in Practice', *Journal of Advanced Nursing*, vol. 2 (1977), p. 111-26; Graham, *The First Months of Motherhood*; Spencer, 'The Identification and Management of Illness by Parents of Young Children'; Perkins, 'Antenatal Care and Postnatal

Nursing: Aspects of the Role of the Midwife in Health Education'; Perkins, 'Having a Baby: An Educational Experience?'.

17. J.W. Lawton and K.F. Shortridge, 'Protective Factors in Human Breast Milk and Colostrum', *Lancet*, vol. 1 (January 1977), p. 253.

18. K.S. McKean, J.D. Baum and K.D. Sloper, 'Factors Influencing Breast Feeding', *Archives of Disease in Childhood*, vol. 50, no. 3 (March 1975), pp. 165-70.

19. Martin, *Infant Feeding 1975: Attitudes and Practice in England and Wales*.

20. Evidence for mothers experiencing difficulty with the medical services can be found in the following studies: J. Lennane and J. Lennane, *Hard Labour* (Gollancz, London, 1974); A. Oakley, *Becoming a Mother* (Martin Robertson, Oxford, 1979); Perkins, 'Having a Baby: An Educational Experience?'; Spencer, 'The Identification and Management of Illness by Parents of Young Children'.

21. G.W. Brown, 'Social Causes of Disease' in D. Tuckett (ed.), *An Introduction to Medical Sociology* (Tavistock, London, 1967); K.J. Roghmann and R.J. Haggerty, 'Daily Stress, Illness and Use of Health Services in Young Families', *Paediatric Research*, vol. 7 (1973), pp. 520-6.

22. Graham, *The First Months of Motherhood*.

23. G. Chamberlain and S. Chave, 'Antenatal Education', *Community Health (Bristol)*, vol. 9 (1977), p. 11.

5 PARENTCRAFT: CONTINUITY AND CHANGE

Professional Traditions and Social Change

Classes for expectant parents, variously known as parentcraft, mother-craft, preparation for parenthood, relaxation classes, or childbirth classes, are now arranged by most Area Health Authorities[1] and are an accepted part of health service provision in Britain. The Court Report on Child Health Services recorded professional enthusiasm for parent-craft classes, but commented:

> Unfortunately we could find little . . . evidence that their content had been systematically constructed. *In view of the importance of the subject we would like to see further study of this aspect of pre-natal care aimed at providing those involved with clearer guidance both on what advice parents need during the antenatal period and how best to give it to them.*[2] (Emphasis as in the original.)

This chapter is concerned with the construction of parentcraft pro-grammes, and the extent to which the pressures which have shaped programmes in the past are relevant to the needs of parents in the present. Influences on the programme offered may, in principle, come either from the professionals who teach, or from the members of the group who come to learn. The stronger of these two influences is likely to be the professional one, and it is therefore appropriate first to examine the traditions of teaching associated with the health service groups involved.

Staff who teach in classes are generally midwives or health visitors; hospital classes may also involve physiotherapists. For these three groups of practitioners teaching is an integral part of their work, whether they teach organised classes or individuals. They have thus developed areas of particular interest and concern, which can usefully be treated as two separate traditions; these will be referred to as the midwifery and health visiting traditions. The midwifery tradition, rooted in the sole responsibility of the midwife for the care and comfort of women in normal labour, gave rise to teaching which aimed to reduce women's fear of childbirth, and provided some self-help methods to cope with pain. More recently, obstetric physiotherapists, with their special expertise in self-help methods, have contributed to this tradition. The second tradition may be called the health visiting tradition, and derives from the original role of the health visitor as 'sanitary missioner' to the poor, improving hygiene and nutrition. Classes stemming from this tradition concentrated on child care. It is now rare to find NHS classes concentrating exclusively on either labour or child care, and both midwives and health visitors are involved in both sorts of teaching. Nevertheless, the influence of the two traditions persists in existing programmes.

The professional groups with which these traditions may be associated have themselves changed considerably since classes were made generally available after World War II. The drive towards 100 per cent hospital delivery has broken the continuity of care which was once available from the community midwifery service. The development of antenatal care, with its attendant technology and medical involvement, has led to its concentration either in GPs' antenatal clinics or in hospitals. In either type of clinic, the situation demands some organisation, and hospital clinics in particular encourage the task-oriented type of care where women progress from one person interested in blood to another interested in blood pressure. Where women are delivered in hospital, they tend to receive at least some postnatal care on the wards, and again there is a strong temptation to go for efficiency at the expense of care for the individual.[3] While hospital delivery and technical antenatal care may have contributed to safety for mother and baby, they raise considerable problems for the teaching role of the midwife.

Midwives who knew their patients well could explain things as they went along, could guess at areas of ignorance and misunderstanding, and if they guessed wrong had plenty of opportunities to find out and do better next time. Teaching patients could thus be a natural continuation of care. Now that many midwives see a woman during her pregnancy mainly in the context of an antenatal clinic, which may well not be conducive to relaxed conversation, either teaching may be neglected, or it may be felt to be a rather artificial process, disrupting the smooth flow of activity in the clinic, needing careful organisation and, perhaps, better done somewhere else.

Home visits by community midwives may seem to be one solution. Yet most women in their first pregnancy are likely to be at work in the daytime, at least until they are 28 weeks pregnant; frequent home visits to all such mothers in the evening are probably beyond the capabilities of the most dedicated community midwives at present staffing levels. After all, they have other work to do as well. If clinics and home visits have limitations, because of pressure of other work, it could be argued

that antenatal classes provide a solution to midwives' difficulties in
teaching women during pregnancy, or worse still, perhaps, on busy
labour wards.[4] Gathering women together in antenatal classes could
seem to be more efficient, with one midwife teaching twelve women,
instead of one to one. It even gives staff the opportunity to teach husbands, who are likely to be absent from antenatal clinics, and from the
home during daytime visits in pregnancy, and thus inaccessible to direct
professional influence. Antenatal classes seem to solve the professional
problems of access and lack of time, at least in relation to those women
and their partners who attend such classes. They may also be seen as
easing the problems of complexity of material which face midwives
trying to explain about antenatal checks and labour ward technology.
At least in an organised class the teacher can prepare an explanation,
possibly with suitable visual aids, and spend time on dealing with questions without worrying about the queue forming in the waiting area.
Seeing classes as at least a partial solution to midwives' professional
problems may encourage them to add many items to the programme of
antenatal classes.

Health visitors have different problems, but similar pressures still
exist. The chronic under-staffing of the health visiting service[5] creates
permanent conflict for health visitors trained and expecting to be
'family visitors'.[6] Torn between their traditional preoccupation with
mothers and small children, and the new pressures towards involvement
with the rest of the population, usually increased by their attachment
to general practitioners, they frequently have difficulty in making as
many home visits as they would like. They also face the difficulty of
deciding whether to concentrate their help on a few problem families,
or whether to spread their attention among the more capable families
who could still use their help. Antenatal classes may seem to be a good
place to provide information on solid foods, immunisation, toilet
training and child development, so that parents will not go without this
information because the health visitor cannot visit regularly.

The two major professional traditions encourage the running of
classes; these traditions, together with major changes in professional
practice, have influenced the programme which is presented to parents.
Arguments from professional convenience, however, are not sufficient
justification for a teaching programme. It is also necessary to show that
what is offered is appropriate to the situation of the learner, or the
learning group, and related to their problems as well as to those of the
professionals. Before moving on to look at the programme in more
detail, it is worth remembering that changes have taken place in society

as well as in professional practice, and examining the effects of these changes on the transition to parenthood.

Having babies and rearing children has become more complex, since the choices open to parents have increased in number. Effective contraception has given couples the choice of whether to have children and increased the psychological importance of following through this choice by bringing the child up well. The choices of place of delivery and type of pain relief available to modern women in childbirth were far more restricted 30 years ago. Social and geographical mobility bring young couples into contact with many different ways of bringing up children. People now argue about whether babies should be fed on demand; whether — and when — children should be left to cry; and at what age it is possible, or desirable, to punish a child, for what acts. With increased choice in these matters come the drawbacks. Efficient contraception means that there are fewer babies around to watch half-consciously, or care for occasionally, before starting a family. A new mother can feel relieved that 'since Mum isn't round the corner, I don't have to stop her interfering', but on the other hand 'she isn't there when I need her, and who *can* I get to help with the baby?'

In addition, the standards of performance are higher. It is no longer enough for parents to raise a healthy child, an achievement in itself when infant mortality was higher and childbirth more dangerous. Now parents are likely to be blamed, and to blame themselves, for any problems with a child's emotional, intellectual and moral development. The issue of discipline is a good illustration of the problems parents face; everyone agrees it is important, but it is by no means agreed whether a well-disciplined child obeys without arguing, or obeys when given a reason. Nor is it agreed how the results are to be achieved.[7] All that is clear is that an ill-disciplined child is a nuisance and the 'fault' of the parents. Life was much simpler when people believed in original sin, that to spare the rod was to spoil the child, and could blame continued obstinacy on his own evil nature if the approved remedy failed to work. Added to the original professional reasons for running classes, therefore, we have the picture of young couples faced with a multiplicity of choices and a shortage of both personal experience and of reliable lay support. This problem is frequently expressed by new parents as 'conflicting advice' and it is not, of course, confined to the neighbours, relatives and friends. Professionals, unfortunately, give conflicting advice as well.[8]

The Present Programme – The Main Emphasis

How far do antenatal classes tackle these problems, professional and social? A survey on hospital and community classes[9] in one Area Health Authority in 1977 provides material to examine this question. Hospital midwives and health visitors were asked to consult their colleagues in physiotherapy and community midwifery where appropriate, and to indicate the length of time spent on particular topics in the antenatal class programme. Seven topics emerged as being the most time-consuming, with the vast majority of classes including these as an important part of their programme: labour, pain relief in labour, a film on the birth of a baby, breast feeding, artificial feeding, bathing a baby and a trip round the local maternity unit (see Table 5.1).

Table 5.1: Main Topics

	Rank Order (27 possible topics)	
	Community Staff (48)	Hospital Staff (5)
Film on birth of baby	1	2[a]
Labour	2	1
Breast feeding	3	4
Class tour of maternity unit	4[a]	5
Artificial feeding	5	7
Bathing a baby	6	3
Pain relief in labour	7	6

[a] Indicates that the topic was omitted by more than ten per cent of the group.

These topics derive from the two health service teaching traditions. From the midwifery tradition comes the high proportion of time devoted to labour, which does not include the physical preparation offered in all these classes, the illustration of labour by a film on birth and the attention to pain relief. The provision of a trip round the maternity hospital shows the adaptation of the midwifery tradition to take account of the trend towards 100 per cent hospital confinement, and the other topics clearly can be taught in such a way as to prepare women for technological childbirth, though, as the material in Chapter 3 shows, this is not always the case.

The legacies of the midwifery tradition, while valuable, are clearly time-consuming. Learning about parenthood, therefore, takes up only a part of the time available in antenatal classes. The legacies of the health visiting tradition, concerned with child care, would seem to be more promising in this context. Feeding the baby successfully is, after all, the most basic task of parents, since if they fail in this task they are unlikely to continue to be parents. In this sense, parenthood has not changed. What has changed is the context in which feeding is carried out. In a social setting where public breast feeding is not common, and many grown women have never seen a baby breast fed, those responsible for antenatal education are urged to teach about breast feeding and encourage mothers to try, on the grounds that it is best for baby. The prominence of breast feeding as a topic on the programme reflects this concern. The topic of artificial feeding relates to both aspects of the health visiting tradition — good food and good hygiene. Classes normally stress the importance of mixing feeds correctly, to avoid the risk of either underfeeding or dehydrating the baby, and the importance of sterilising feeding bottles, to avoid the risk of infection. There are clearly some women who need intensive instruction on mixing feeds and sterilising bottles in order to protect the health or even the lives of their babies.[10] Classes in areas with a high infant mortality rate, like many of our inner cities, will naturally spend time on these topics, even though for some women the early teaching will need to be reinforced by individual sessions in their own homes.

However, it is worth remembering in this context that health visiting is no longer a matter of hygiene inspection and instruction. This change has taken place because it is assumed that the majority of the population no longer *need* instruction in basic hygiene, and are likely to feel insulted if it is offered to them. In view of this change, it is strange to see the persistence of hygiene-based topics in a prominent position on the programme for antenatal classes for a whole Area Health Authority, which is certainly not generally afflicted with the problems of the inner city. While expectant mothers are not necessarily offended by hygiene-based topics when they are about babies, they might well benefit more from an alternative programme of teaching. Baby bathing is, ostensibly, about hygiene and little else. It is commonly taught again on the post-natal wards or by the community midwives, or both. Some mothers find a sense of unreality in the presentation of this topic before the baby has arrived; this is heightened when the teaching session involves bathing a doll, not a live baby.

Q. How much of that child care teaching in classes did you find helpful?

A. Er . . . some of it, the bath part is something they show you again in hospital. I think it is a bit pointless sitting there with a

doll. It's different when you've got a screaming baby. I thought
that was rather a waste of time. It's better to wait 'til you've got
to hospital with nurses there with live babies. Anybody can sit
there and bath a doll y'know, turn it over the right way and
that.[11]

It could be argued that bathing should be taught after the baby has
arrived, when a mother can learn by doing; when this suggestion is
made, some midwives and health visitors argue that the topic is not
really about hygiene at all. They use the session to demonstrate the
features of the newborn infant, or to teach about relationships. Both
these arguments lose most of their force if the 'baby' is in fact a rubber
doll; even if it is a live baby, they neglect the reasonable assumption of
the class that what they are supposed to be learning is what is being
demonstrated — how to bath a baby. Observation of individual classes[12]
suggests that women watch the movements of the teacher as she baths,
and ask questions which relate to the process — how to test the water,
for example. They appear to be trying hard to absorb every detail of a
technical process. Those midwives and health visitors who wish to teach
about relationships by bathing a baby must first overcome their group's
attempts to concentrate on the techniques which they are not, in fact,
supposed to be learning.

The Present Programme — Secondary Professional Interests

The reader will have noted that among the main topics in the programme, none is directly concerned with the issues of expanding choice
and social variation discussed at the beginning of this chapter. Since
each of these main topics could readily occupy one session of a course,
which is normally six to eight sessions with possibly an additional session in the evening, there is not an enormous amount of time left.
Further, there are other topics in the programme too.

Table 5.1, showing main topics, also showed evidence of general
professional agreement. Most midwives and health visitors taught most
of these topics for much the same length of time. Tables 5.2 and 5.3,
however, show wide professional divergence, not only between hospital
and community, but also within the two groups. This is hardly surprising when we look at the topics involved. Midwives and health visitors
in this Area stated that women attending classes were in late pregnancy.[13] Teaching is being provided about what to eat, when the

information is too late to benefit them much if they use it, and about what to buy for the baby, when they have already bought it or been given it. It is not surprising that a proportion of the professionals involved have reduced the amount of time they spend on these topics. What is surprising is that those who have begun to doubt the value of teaching these subjects retain them in an over-crowded programme at all. Similarly, many doubt whether it is appropriate to teach family planning to expectant parents who have their minds on the forthcoming birth, or to tackle the more distant issues of solid foods and immunisations. It will perhaps not surprise some community staff that hospital antenatal classes do not advertise the community services; what should give them pause for thought is that many of their community colleagues doubt the need to explain in any detail how the health visitor and the child health clinic can help new parents.

Table 5.2: Too Late?

| | Rank Order (27 possible topics) | |
	Community Staff (48)	Hospital Staff (5)
The layette	8^a	8
Diet in pregnancy	16^a	9^a
The maternity services – how the system works	19^{ab}	23

a Indicates wide variation in the time spent on these topics.
b Indicates omission of the topic by more than ten per cent of staff.

Table 5.3: Too Soon?

| | Rank Order (27 possible topics) | |
	Community Staff (48)	Hospital Staff (5)
Family planning	9^a	12^a
Introducing solid foods	13^a	
Immunisation	14^a	25^b
Work of health visitor	15^a	26^b
Child health clinic	18^a	24^b

a Indicates wide variation in the time spent on these topics.
b Indicates omission of the topic by more than ten per cent of staff.

These two tables show professionals uncertain, as a body, about what it is appropriate to teach. For some the tradition from which they operate has force; hospital staff with a bias to the midwifery tradition may stress antenatal topics, whereas community staff may be more readily influenced by the health visiting tradition to spend time on solid foods and immunisation. But for neither group do these traditions carry sufficient authority to prevent the doubts of some members being expressed in the limited time they spend on some of these topics. Their relevance to expectant parents at the end of the woman's pregnancy is being questioned.

The Present Programme — Family Topics

Parenthood, it has been argued, is more than child care.[14] The health visiting tradition, within its limitations, provides for child care; it derives, however, from a period when parenthood involved less conscious choice in whether to undertake it and what good child rearing was. When antenatal classes cover topics concerned with family life, they move outside the limits of the two traditions which inspired them, and break new ground. Not surprisingly, there is considerable variation in the process.

Table 5.4: Family Topics

	Rank Order (27 possible topics)	
	Community Staff (48)	Hospital Staff (5)
The family unit	10[b]	10[a]
The child's need for security	11[a]	20[b]
The role of the father	17[a]	11[a]

[a] Indicates wide variation in the time spent on these topics.
[b] Indicates omission of topic by more than ten per cent of staff.

The programme which we have been examining was taught mainly to mothers — thus it was frequently called 'mothercraft'. Fathers were invited to evening meetings during 41 out of 92 community courses, and three out of five hospital courses. It might be expected that with fathers present, more family-based topics would be covered; however, these classes were normally largely taken up by a film, or in some cases a hospital visit, and comparatively few midwives and health visitors were using the time to discuss the choices facing young parents in the way in which they organise their family lives. A few centres were offering 'parentcraft' classes for both parents earlier in pregnancy, but the programme seemed very similar to 'mothercraft', except that 'parentcraft' contained no physical preparation. Even the name, 'parentcraft' is an indicator of an attempted response to social change.

For it is used ambiguously. It may, as in the previous paragraph, be used to distinguish classes for both parents from those for mothers only, a description governed by the recipient of the teaching. It is also used, however, to describe the material taught. Staff who recognise that fathers do look after their babies are uncomfortable with the implications of 'mothercraft' because it suggests that only mothers do these things. Thus 'parentcraft' may be used to describe classes which, in practice, are attended by women only, on the grounds that the skills, if not the classes, are unisex.

The uncertainty shown in Table 5.4 about teaching family topics directly is paralleled by the uneven provision of models from which expectant parents can learn indirectly. If part of the difficulty experienced by many couples with their first child comes from their unfamiliarity with small babies, then antenatal classes could usefully address themselves to this problem. 'Bathing a baby' may be a popular class, at least in prospect, if women believe they will see a real baby, not a doll being bathed. Such an expectation is not necessarily fulfilled; this study of one Area's antenatal class programme showed that only a third of the community classes and one of the five of the hospital classes had a baby to visit them. There is, in any case, a good case for leaving this particular topic out of the programme altogether, to be taught in hospital by community midwives after the baby has arrived.

An alternative class to which mother and baby could usefully be invited is that on breast feeding. Again this was comparatively rare; only a quarter of the community classes and none of the hospital classes did this. Yet a mother who is successfully breast feeding is far superior as a teaching aid to any film or poster. Women used to learn to breast feed by watching other women throughout their early lives, thus needing less skilled help when the baby actually arrived. An antenatal class cannot compensate for the lack of twenty years' experience, but it can at least make a start. A third possibility is to unite the two problems of lack of experience and social change, and invite new parents back with their babies to talk about their own experiences of birth and of adjusting to family life. The antenatal teacher would obviously exercise some care in issuing invitations, but abnormal deliveries, for example, need not be screened out. Forceps deliveries and caesarean sections are well known to exist and it may be reassuring to see that despite a complicated delivery, mother and baby are fine. It may be helpful to invite two couples, so that the different experiences balance one another and the teacher has less need to underline the fact that births, and babies, vary.[15] This sort of class provides both up-to-

date information and an opportunity for expectant parents to identify
with the new parents and to consider the models of parenthood which
they represent. Again, people are far better teaching aids than films.
The characters on film cannot answer questions!

Tradition and Method

This examination of the standard programme in one Area Health
Authority shows the persisting influence of the two traditions of antenatal teaching, and the extent to which their validity as a guide to programme content was being questioned by the midwives and health
visitors most directly involved. It would be unjust to dismiss this Area
as a backwater, years behind the times.[16] For example, the Salop programme, formulated in 1974, was published in 1975 in instalments in
the *Midwives' Chronicle and Nursing Notes*,[17] a journal where one
might reasonably expect to find professional traditions well expressed.
This programme lasts seven weeks, and no detail is given on the stage of
pregnancy of the women for whom it is intended; in the absence of
specific information it is reasonable to assume that women will come
when it is most convenient to them, that is, for first-time mothers, at
28 weeks or later, when most will finish work. The first two sessions of
this programme cover maternity benefits, 'Shopping for baby and you',
antenatal care, smoking, drugs and diet in pregnancy, and minor dis-
orders in pregnancy. Much of this material is fairly irrelevant *to women
in late pregnancy*. It should be covered in early pregnancy when acting
on advice will bring benefit, and information can prevent worry. The
absence from the Salop programme of any exploration of the relationship between stage of pregnancy and material taught parallels the
willingness of midwives and health visitors in the Area studied to retain
topics in the programme about which there was clearly considerable
professional uncertainty.

Women in late pregnancy are hardly physically unobtrusive. No
trained professional could possibly be in doubt; staff have only to look
at their group to see that the women before them will deliver in two or
three months' time. So why do so few of them act on their observations
in relation to the programme they teach? One reason is that tradition
has power over more than content; it also influences method. Tables
5.1, 5.2 and 5.3 are full of topics which lend themselves readily to a
teacher telling a group about them, or showing a film which does it for
her. The professional knows the facts about labour, diet in pregnancy,

solid foods, or whatever. While she stays within the tradition, her only problem is 'putting it over', which usually means having the nerve to stand up in front of a group, keeping going, and having suitable visual aids to emphasise or illustrate what she is saying. Craven, Crouch and Goosey of Salop AHA point out that, 'Many of us are reluctant to stand up and speak in front of others; we are shy and perhaps lacking in confidence'. This is both true and sympathetic. In their use of the phrase 'speak in front of', it is also entirely traditional. Teaching, here, is telling. A variant on this approach shifts the emphasis from speaking to doing things in front of a group — the demonstration. Here the teacher shows the group a procedure; for example, mixing feeds, sterilising bottles, bathing a baby. This method has its roots in nursing procedure, and midwives and health visitors will no doubt draw on their own experience of being shown how to do things, as they will on their experience of being told about things. Here, indeed, parentcraft is parent *craft*.

Neither telling nor demonstrating are suitable teaching methods for family topics, as they have been described here, and this is one of the reasons for the massive professional uncertainty about handling them shown in Table 5.4. Midwives and health visitors cannot be insulated from the general uncertainty about the proper roles of husband and wife, or mother and father; many will be working out in their own families the implications of working mothers for the role of fathers. Health visitors, in their professional capacity, see every day the varieties of ways in which parents can bring up children. Many of those teaching antenatal classes will have developed strong personal views on certain aspects of family life; they are also likely to be well aware that their views are not generally accepted. If they retain the traditional method of telling things to groups, while trying to move away from the traditional content, they are likely to find themselves pushing their own opinions at a group which may well not share them. It is right that staff should be wary of this.

One way of expressing this wariness is to spend as little time as possible on these difficult topics. This seems to have been the solution adopted by many of the staff in the study area, as the variation in Table 5.4 suggests. It is also the solution apparently preferred by Salop AHA. The programme features a class entitled 'Happy Families', which includes: the health visitor's job description, child health clinics, developmental checks, immunisation, and weaning, minor problems of management in the first few months, safety in the home, contraception and the postnatal examination, as well as 'marital relations', and a section headed:

Planning the Day
To suit husband and wife. Tolerance and humour will be necessary.
Housework; rest; meals; social life; baby sitter; grannies. Emotional
instability; jealousy; husband; children; animals!

Clearly not much time can be available for these somewhat complicated
topics.

An alternative to this approach is to teach about family life or
relationships indirectly. Baby bathing is sometimes justified as indirect
teaching about relationships. Yet the baby, if it appears in person at
all, is usually bathed by the professional in charge, not by its mother or
father. The baby has no relationship with the professional, and may
howl pitifully throughout to underline the fact. Parents are more likely
to learn about relationships by watching mother and baby reunited. If
this is the object of the class, why separate them in the first place? This
convoluted way of teaching about relationships, with all the complications for the group in working out what they are supposed to be
attending to, could surely be improved. A third solution to the problem
of family topics lies in incidental teaching, slipping in odd comments on
relationships in the course of talks on other topics, such as 'don't let
the baby take over your life', or 'men are no good with small babies'.[18]
This solution carries with it two risks. For the couple, or the woman,
who has already developed strong views about child-centred child
rearing or husband involvement in child care, comments like this may
be infuriating, all the more so because they are asides to the main purpose of the class, and thus cannot easily be argued about. For the
couple, or the woman, who has not yet developed clear ideas,
comments like this may come over with the full force of professional
authority, which is not justifiable and may not have been intended.
Ways of adapting to the new baby, and the part which fathers can play
in child care are open questions which need full discussion, not premature solutions in one sentence from a professional.

The Public Image of the Teacher

Traditional content and traditional method thus dovetail together to
make a unified whole, and tackling the awkward topics concerned with
modern family life means that professional staff must look outside the

traditions for help with method as well as content. Since midwives and health visitors are *teaching*, the obvious place for them to look is to the teaching profession for models. This is unlikely to be reassuring. The last thing an antenatal group should look like is a school classroom, particularly a school classroom of fifteen or more years ago, which is what most midwives and health visitors will remember from their own experience. School teachers, for this generation, are unlikely to provide an alternative model, merely a slicker version of their own efforts. Teachers, as we all believed at infant school, know everything; they are competent, organised, poised, can handle every situation that comes up — and, of course, they are never nervous. This stereotype, inaccurate though every teacher knows it to be, is readily available and potentially damaging to the self-confidence of those who take it seriously as an ideal for which they should be aiming.

It is also very unhelpful to anyone trying to deal with topics to which no one has final answers. A midwife or health visitor might say 'If teachers know everything then surely I ought to know the answers on subjects put on the programme?' The acceptance that teachers never do know everything and that therefore midwives and health visitors acting as teachers need not pretend to do so either, makes it easier to look for information, and insights, from the group, and to leave open questions open. Helping people to talk about problems, and thus come nearer to their own solutions, may be easier for health service staff to approach through their existing expertise in work with individual patients, rather than through reference to their own experience of the education system.

Nevertheless, antenatal classes are about teaching, and midwives and health visitors have professional expertise to offer. They know a lot about the process of adapting to family life, and they can offer their experience for others to use. For example, instead of 'don't let the baby take over your life' as a sideline on feeding, the midwife or health visitor can comment in the course of a discussion that total and unremitting devotion to the interests of the baby is likely to leave a mother drained, tense and eventually unable to care for it properly. Thus planning some time for rest and relaxation is a good idea, for the baby's sake as well as her own and her husband's. The point is made from professional expertise, but it is a contribution to a couple's decision-making, not an attempt to pre-empt it.

Why Change?

Antenatal teachers within the health service are thus working within the confines of fairly powerful traditions, which retain their force because part of these traditions are still appropriate. They may also be reinforced from outside if there is management pressure to stick to a prescribed programme – or, perhaps more important, if teaching staff believe that there is such pressure. They may well lack alternative models of what classes could look like if they did not consist of a teacher telling the group, and the group asking questions within the limits of what is apparently relevant that week. In this situation it is most encouraging to see that change is, nevertheless, taking place, though rather unevenly and slowly. One stimulus for this may be personal to individual staff; a dislike of being lectured at may lead them to decide not to lecture others if at all possible, and to experiment with alternative methods. Another stimulus is the existence of increasingly vocal consumer groups related to the health service. It is difficult now to escape from the idea that professionals are not always and invariably right about what patients, or clients, want or need. Not everyone wishes to apply this uncomfortable notion to their own practice, but for those who do, it encourages doubts about the validity of the traditional programme.

Reconsideration of content and method for this reason would be easier for professionals if expectant parents, or perhaps particularly expectant mothers, were less docile, and less willing to accept the programme provided without suggesting improvements. Groups which soak up all that is given to them, because their members are too unsure of themselves to put forward views about what they want, provide little stimulus to a teacher. Where those responsible for teaching are continuously offering short courses, covering the same ground every six or eight weeks, they may readily become bored, and, in time, boring. In this atmosphere it is easy for the traditional programme to be taught in the traditional way until no one quite remembers who planned it, or why. In addition, the problems of establishing what expectant parents need is bedevilled by timing; if they are asked before the birth, they may not know enough to be at all specific about what they want; if they are asked afterwards, the chances are that their priorities have changed, and they are preoccupied with baby care rather than with labour. Asking the consumer, while an interesting exercise and one which may well yield useful insights,[19] is no substitute for professional thought and experiment.

Experiment will have to be in method as well as in content. Methods which implicitly restrict questions to those directly relevant to the topic of the day will not help practitioners to see whether there are other things that the group would like to talk about. Teaching practical skills may readily have this effect; so may methods which rely heavily on telling, particularly at the beginning of a course where the tone is set for the rest. 'The layette' would surely not have persisted so long as an important topic in the antenatal class programme in late pregnancy if teachers had asked the group to talk about what they had bought, and to pass on tips to one another about cheap nappies, etc., instead of professionals doing most of the talking themselves. The experimental antenatal teacher must listen as well as talk, so that she can pick up hints of what concerns her particular group and adjust either her pro-gramme, or her line of approach to a topic, accordingly. As one mother commented:

I think rather than talk blindly on, they ought to let people ask. You go in, and they give a talk, very helpful really, but they might put you on a subject, or a small item, that will trigger something off and you sit and think 'shall I ask, because I've got that'. At the end they say 'any questions' and they sit looking at one another, and I think that instead of them sitting talking they ought to let you all talk, because it is then that you spill your fears.[20]

Notes

1. A.E. Brammer, 'Report of an Enquiry into Organised Classes for Pregnant Women and their Partners Provided by the Maternity Services in England in 1975', unpublished report (Royal College of Midwives, London, 1977).

2. Report of the Committee on Child Health Services, *Fit for the Future* (HMSO, London, 1976).

3. Elizabeth R. Perkins, 'Antenatal Care and Postnatal Nursing: Aspects of the Role of the Midwife in Health Education' in D.C. Anderson (ed.), *Health Education in Practice* (Croom Helm, London, 1979).

4. See Chapter 2.

5. Report of the Committee on Child Health Services, *Fit for the Future*, recorded that health visiting strength was 50 per cent below that recommended by the Jameson Committee in 1956, and restated by the DHSS in 1972.

6. Report of a Working Party on the Field of Work, Training and Recruitment of Health Visitors, 'An Enquiry into Health Visiting' (Ministry of Health, London, 1950).

7. For a further exploration of the differences between social groups on these and other issues, see in particular the works of John and Elizabeth Newson, *Patterns of Infant Care in an Urban Community* (1963), *Four Years Old in an Urban Community* (1968), and *Seven Years Old in the Home Environment*

(1976) (Allen & Unwin, London).

8. Gaynor D. Maclean, 'An Appraisal of the Concepts of Infant Feeding and their Application in Practice', *Journal of Advanced Nursing*, vol. 2 (1977), pp. 111-26; Elizabeth R. Perkins, 'Having a Baby: An Educational Experience?', Occasional Paper 6 (Leverhulme Health Education Project, University of Nottingham, 1978); N.J. Spencer, 'The Identification and Management of Illness by Parents of Young Children', unpublished MPhil thesis, University of Nottingham, presented 1980.

9. Further details of the methods used are available in Elizabeth R. Perkins, 'Defining the Need: An Analysis of Varying Teaching Goals in Antenatal Classes', *International Journal of Nursing Studies*, vol. 16 (1979), pp. 275-82.

10. J.A.D. Anderson and A. Gatherer, 'Hygiene of Infant Feeding Utensils: Practice and Standards in the Home', *British Medical Journal*, vol. 2 (1970), pp. 20-3; B. Owen and M. Portress, 'Prospective Investigation into Cot Deaths', *Health Visitor*, vol. 48 (October 1975), p. 379.

11. This quotation is drawn from material collected by Dr S. Packer and Miss S. Snell; details of the study are available in Perkins, 'Antenatal Care and Post-natal Nursing: Aspects of the Role of the Midwife in Health Education'; or in Perkins, 'Having a Baby: An Educational Experience?'.

12. Elizabeth R. Perkins, 'Parentcraft: A Comparative Study of Teaching Method', Occasional Paper 16 (Leverhulme Health Education Project, University of Nottingham, 1979).

13. Perkins, 'Defining the Need: An Analysis of Varying Teaching Goals in Antenatal Classes'.

14. Esther M. Goody, 'Parental Roles in Anthropological Perspective', in DHSS, *The Family and Society: Dimensions of Parenthood* (HMSO, London, 1974).

15. For more details of what this might look like, see Perkins, 'Parentcraft: A Comparative Study of Teaching Method'.

16. The programme has, in addition, been revised since the study was completed, partly as a result of the study.

17. R.O. Craven, M. Crouch and R.A. Goosey, 'Guidelines for Teachers of Parentcraft and Relaxation', *Midwives' Chronicle and Nursing Notes* (January-August, 1975).

18. These comments are actual, not imaginary; see Perkins, 'Parentcraft: A Comparative Study of Teaching Method'.

19. See, for example, the useful and thought-provoking material in A.C. Breese, 'Antenatal Classes and Preparation for Pregnancy, Birth and Mother-hood', unpublished MMedSci dissertation, University of Nottingham, 1976.

20. See note 11.

6 RESPONDING TO GROUPS: TOWARDS BETTER ANTENATAL TEACHING

The Freedom to Ask Questions

It has been argued in Chapter 5 that the teaching style adopted by
many health service group teachers limits their capacity to identify and
respond to the group's needs, and to tackle new subjects with imagina-
tion. This argument would be (and, indeed, in my experience has been)
indignantly rejected by some midwives and health visitors who teach
groups. 'Our groups', they say 'are very informal. People are free to ask
questions at any time. Certainly we don't talk all the time. You've been
watching all the wrong people at work.' Now of course no generalisa-
tion can possibly apply to every individual, and indeed there are also
health service teachers who are skilled in responding to the needs of a
group. But some of those who reject this analysis are in fact failing to
distinguish between responding to individual, clearly articulated needs
expressed in questions on the topic in hand, or not too far away from it,
and being willing to work with the group to help them to identify their
own needs, and to meet them. It is worth repeating here part of the
comment of the lady who wanted 'more discussion', quoted at the end
of Chapter 5: 'I think that instead of them sitting talking they ought to
let you all talk, because it is then that you spill your fears.'
   She understood the difference between asking questions and 'spilling
your fears'. And, as I argued in Chapter 3, until some of those fears are
expressed, a teacher's attempt to reassure may in fact do damage, by
tackling the wrong fear in the wrong way. Failing to assess and respond
to group needs does not necessarily indicate an insensitive or authoritarian personality. It merely suggests an absence of the appropriate
technique. To illustrate this, and other technical points in this chapter,
extracts from transcripts of antenatal classes will be used. These classes
were each taught by a midwife and health visitor working together. The
transcripts and the analysis have been made with their help, providing
insights which only they could give. The selection of particular passages
to illustrate particular points inevitably involves some distortion of
their individual teaching styles, and I am grateful to them for allowing
me to do this.[1] A list of symbols used in transcription can be found at
the end of this chapter.
   The distinction between answering questions and encouraging discus-

sion is rooted in a distinction between responding to individuals and responding to groups. This extract shows a community midwife (MW) at the end of a talk on the advantages, disadvantages and process of breast feeding. She and her colleague are pressed for time; they intend to cover bottle feeding in this session as well, and must finish on time since some of the group have small children to pick up from school. The professionals have therefore *planned* the session with tight timing, and this is reflected in what the midwife says. This extract starts with her final comments on the importance of rest for successful breast feeding, and goes on to outline what the professionals intend to happen next:

Transcript 1

13.1 MW   if you don't get enough rest you won't make the milk —
           you'll be building up tension in yourself and it's just a
           vicious circle — you know so those are the three main
           things that you've got to concentrate on till till you get a
           good supply of milk and you've established good breast
           feeding (4.0) er — I think that's all I'll talk about at the
           moment — with breast feeding (1.0) er — and then Jenny
           can talk about bottle feeding — and then we'll go over a
           few different subjects —

13.2 Mrs S Could I just ask what you said about adequate fluids
            because don't you remember last time somebody said oh
            you don't really need to drink any extra but on reflec-
            tion since I don't think I drink very much *anyway* so
            (probably) I should have been drinking more —

13.3 MW   Sometimes you er — you automatically drink more
            because your body needs it — some people say well I am
            drinking a lot — it's because your body's asking for it —
            you know because you're breast feeding —

13.4 Mrs S But if you don't feel the need to drink any more then
            you're probably all right —

13.5 HV   I think that was probably — I think I was talking to you
            about this because we were a little bit worried

14.1   whether Matthew was getting enough weren't we and
            think you were er — drinking rather a lot and there is a
            theory that if you drink *wildly* in excess of your needs
            that it can wash away the hormone that makes the
            milk —

14.2 Mrs S That's what I understood —

14.3 HV   And I think it may be in your case I wondered if you
            were doing this — in fact Matthew did start to gain
            weight soon after that but he was perfectly happy
            although he hadn't actually regained his birth weight for
            three weeks had he —
14.4 Mrs S No —
14.5 HV   I can remember that — we did have a long discussion
            about that and whether you know you were taking per-
            haps a little bit too much er — in excess of your needs —
14.6 Mrs S So much happened since I suppose that I don't remem-
            ber all the details — I just — it just sticks in my mind
            that you said that you probably don't need to drink
            more and since I've thought about I think (I'd do better)
            (   ) (milk) (1.0)
14.7 HV   Because fluid requirements do vary a great deal — you
            know it is a fact that we have to make sure you are
            having enough particularly at the beginning I think this
            was you know three weeks on wasn't it when I was er —
            visiting you then and (Matthew) quite happy waking the
            morning with smiles — yes and so er (doctor and I deci-
            ded) he certainly *was* getting enough because I think he
            was growing —
14.8 Mrs S Yes that's right (4.0)

The midwife has not suggested that anyone should ask questions; she
has, if anything, suggested that they should not ask questions: 'I think
that's all I'll talk about at the moment — with breast feeding (1.0) er —
and then Jenny can talk about bottle feeding — and then we'll go over a
few different subjects —'. She makes it clear that there is a full agenda,
and that she and her colleague have a lot to tell them. Nevertheless, Mrs
S asks a question, and the way it is handled is instructive. She is allowed
to expand it — no one interrupts her after, say, 'adequate fluids', with
an answer before she has made the context of her problem clear. The
midwife begins to offer a general answer (13.3), and Mrs S is given time
to rephrase it for herself to make sure she has understood (13.4). At
13.5, the health visitor, knowing the background from which the question has sprung (she was given a clue to this by Mrs S in 13.2 and has
used it to think back), explains why the issue of adequate fluids was
raised with the last baby, provides Mrs S with the details she needs to
explain her memories, which are not very clear (14.6) and, with any
luck, stops her worrying about the problem. This is an excellent

example both of good team teaching and of responding to an individual, particular worry, without rush, without dismissiveness and
without ridicule. This is what many antenatal teachers have in mind
when they say that their groups are free to raise anything, and do. In
itself, it is admirable, and, in addition, shows the advantages of the
distinctive health service combination of care and education in meeting
individual need.

However, we have not exhausted the possibilities of this extract yet.
Mrs S already has one child, Matthew, and it is her experience with
Matthew on which she is drawing for her question. 'Adequate fluids'
was a phrase used by the midwife just before this extract started, and it
could have reminded Mrs S of the problem she had had previously. She
is able to formulate her question reasonably precisely, possibly because
of her past experience. She can thus help the midwife and health visitor
to give her an answer which appears to satisfy her. Not only does she
have her own experience with Matthew on which to draw, she also has
experience of the professional staff who are teaching her now. She
knows that they have helped and supported her during problems with
Matthew and can have an entirely reasonable expectation that they will
help her now. When we add to all that the fact that Mrs S also has a
professional background, it is not at all surprising that she is prepared to
disregard the midwife's discouragement of questions at the end of 13.1.
She has two sets of experience and a reasonable amount of social competence to help her take a very small risk of disapproval from midwife
or health visitor for disrupting the smooth flow of the session.

However, antenatal classes are not composed entirely of women like
Mrs S. This particular class was unusual in having a majority (4:3) of
women having a second baby, and these four women used this session
to ask questions, along the lines that Mrs S does here. Of those expecting
their first baby, only one said anything at all, and all but one of her
comments continued someone else's question on antenatal appointments which was raised before the main subject of feeding had started.
Because these three women said nothing, or practically nothing, it is
impossible, without further conversation with them, for anyone to tell
whether they understood what they were told, let alone whether it met
their needs. There are certainly explanations for their silence, and that
of other silent people in other groups, which are based on personal
characteristics. Some people are shy; some are not very well educated;
some are not very intelligent; some are nervous about asking vague,
poorly formulated questions in front of other people in case they look
stupid. So there may be a small queue of people wanting to have a quiet

word with the midwife or the health visitor at the end of a session. Undoubtedly there are some topics which are private, and women who wish for privacy should not feel forced to discuss their problems in front of a group. But a queue of people should give a teacher pause. It does mean that she is trusted to respond to individual specific problems, as the midwife and health visitor did in the extract, and this is good. However, it may also suggest that the group session has left a lot of problems unsolved and unrecognised by the teacher, and this may not be so good. The explanation for the silence during the group session and the queue following it lies not only in individual women's personalities but also in the way in which the group is handled.

The Crucial Issue of 'Pitch'

What alternatives are there for this session of feeding, with the disturbing division between experienced mothers with queries to raise, and inexperienced mothers, for whom the class could be seen to be primarily intended, with nothing to say for themselves? It is, of course, quite possible that these three ladies understood everything and went away with food for thought. An experienced teacher may develop a sensitivity to the mood of her group that is a good guide to whether she is making real contact. Such a teacher, however, is unlikely to trust her sensitivity alone, as a substitute for explicit response from the group. Insensitive or inexperienced teachers may think they are making contact, whereas in fact one or more of their class are feeling like this woman (who did *not* attend the class featured in Transcript 1).

Transcript 2

Mrs T   Well I think the ones at the — at the relaxation classes are inclined to be a bit of a nuisance because — they only sort of centre on one thing and that was breast feeding — you know they didn't sort of go on to anything else — to me they always seemed to centre on breast feeding all the while you know whether you wanted to do it or not — that's what I — I didn't find them all that helpful — only apart from the — the exercises you know

Interviewer   You think they overdid the bit about breast feeding

Mrs T   Yeh — I think they do a little bit yeh — 'cos I didn't go this time (   )

Interviewer   Er — had you — had you not felt that they overdid the
              breast feeding would you have been more inclined to
              go with this one
Mrs T   Yeh — I think so yeh
Interviewer   They put you off a bit did they
Mrs T   Yeh because they kept drumming it into me you see —
              oh — your child's a lot healthier if you breast feed you
              know and — you can bring them up a lot better if you
              breast feed than what you can on bottles but I — to me
              I don't see that it — makes any difference you know —
              I can't sort of understand why is a baby better brought
              up on breast feeding than what it is on a bottle — you
              know — to me they sort of get the same symptoms —
              as what they would on a bottle where on a bottle *you*
              can eat anything and *do* anything but when you breast
              feed you've got to watch what you eat because of the
              baby — I've had it drummed into me that much that it
              put me right off it — you know I had no feeling to do
              it and I think if *you* don't feel like doing it it's no good
              to the baby anyway 'cos you're not going to be inter-
              ested while you're doing it[2]

One technique which can help to solve the teaching problems both
of the inexperienced, non-contributing, parent and of the parent with
strong existing views of emotional blocks is that of 'pitch'. Antenatal
classes are mixed in ability, age, social class, and experience of parenthood, and increasingly include both sexes. Midwives and health visitors
are aware of this and worry about it, but often fail to take action which
will help them to 'pitch' their talk to the level of the group before
them. Some means of assessing the level of the group before they start
would improve their ability to meet the needs of those before them,
particularly those needs which are not yet clearly defined by the
individuals concerned.

Let us therefore look at the beginning of this session on feeding. A
short 'any questions' period finishes with advice from the midwife not
to go to two or three antenatal appointments in one week, whatever has
happened to the booking system, but to change one appointment when
necessary. The midwife winds up this topic at 4.5 and 4.7 and starts to
talk about feeding:

Transcript 1

4.5 MW   Whenever you can fit it in — you know make sure
somebody's seeing you each week — that's the main
thing — it doesn't really matter you know as long as
either the hospital or the doctor or myself you know —
or whichever you want to come to — make sure you
see someone each week but *don't* come to two or three
in one week

4.6 Mrs C   No

4.7 MW   It would be a bit much for you — right (2.0) right I
think we'd better on about — we're going to talk about
feeding — who's made their minds up definitely what
they're going to do — I hope nobody's definite
((laughter)) (1.0) what are you going to do —

4.8 Mrs A   I'm going to breast feed (   ) —

4.9 Mrs B   Bottle feed

4.10 Mrs C   (I'm going to try and breast feed)

4.11 Mrs S   Breast feed —

4.12 Mrs R   Breast feed —

4.13 MW   Good — the others haven't made their minds up —
good — I think that's the best thing actually — you
know because you you can be swayed one way or
another at the last minute — you know so I think it's
best to leave your mind open — you know just little
things that crop up that might make you change your
mind *one* way or the other but you must remember in
the end that it's your decision — you know and
nobody's going to force you — one way or the other —

5.1   we'll put all the pros and cons before you and then it's
up to you to make what you think (of the results)
either way — but don't think anybody's going to force
you one way or the other — you just think things very
carefully and think what's best for your (baby) — um
— I'm going to talk about — breast feeding and Jenny's
going to talk about bottle feeding — and then you can
decide for yourselves ((laughter))

This extract shows a nodding acquaintance with the idea of pitch.
The midwife has thought to ask before she started what the women are
planning to do; she gets answers from the four experienced mothers,
and from one of the inexperienced mothers, at 4.10. It is interesting to

note that the answer of Mrs C is less clearly audible than the other
four (indicated by brackets round the phrase) and is also more tentatively phrased: 'I'm going to *try* and breast feed' (my emphasis). The
other two inexperienced mothers say nothing; the midwife takes it that
they are undecided, possibly responding to non-verbal clues, and
follows this by suggesting that indecision is perfectly acceptable, and
indeed, a good idea at this stage. What she does not do is to check on
whether she is right in her guess, or her interpretation of a shrug, and
these two really are undecided. It could be, after all, that they have
heard that midwives and health visitors are in favour of breast feeding
and are scared to say that the whole idea makes them feel sick. One
way to explore this issue immediately would be to ask them what they
have heard and thought about it. Instead of continuing, as in 5.1, 'um
— I'm going to talk about breast feeding . . .' and then going on to
explain her views on the advantages and disadvantages of breast feeding
and bottle feeding, it would have been possible to say instead 'What
have people told you already about feeding methods?' 'Do you have
friends who've breast fed, or bottle fed? What did they say?' 'Have you
talked about it with your husband at all? Your mother?' Any of these
questions, and plenty more, are possible ways of getting started with
the two who have apparently not decided. Those who have decided can
be brought in more readily and asked for their reasons; those who have
already had babies can contribute to a discussion of advantages, disadvantages and solutions to social problems. Here one of the experienced mothers is apparently trying to give her own experience:

Transcript 1

5.1 MW   — if you go out anywhere you haven't got to bother
             about packing it up in a picnic case or anything and in
             fact sterilizing everything — you can just *go* where you
             want and feed — and you'll find now that the way of
             life in the past few years has altered — you know all
             the time and even in — if you want to go shopping or
             anything —

5.2 Mrs A   I think the breast feed problem is to go shopping —

5.3 MW   Well there *are* certain places in *** that do er — pro-
             vide places for you to breast feed your baby like in **
             now they do have a little room that (you can take)
             babies to breast feed —

The midwife, however, is under way with her own explanation and cuts her short. She does not develop a discussion out of her sensible start; by not doing so she reduces the chance of pitching the rest of the session at the right level, because she and her colleague are deprived of the information a discussion would have given them. They have also lost the best chance of getting the inexperienced mothers to talk during this session, since an early discussion on advantages and disadvantages would ask from them only that they should contribute some of their own uncertainties — which the midwife has already made clear are natural and even desirable at this stage. Later in the session, when the talk turns on the technicalities of breast feeding and bottle feeding, they could well have felt that they would look foolish if they asked questions because they had not understood. If they had broken the ice by talking at the beginning, they would have found this risk easier to take.

It is worth emphasising that setting up such a discussion does not mean that a teacher abdicates and ceases to teach. She will make direct contributions to the discussion based on her own expertise, as do other members of the group. Her expertise here will be professional, concerned with such technical matters as antibodies in colostrum; she can wait to see whether other people have expertise on social problems such as breast feeding while shopping. If she has experienced mothers in her group who have breast fed before, some solutions should be available from them, and she can use a different sort of professional expertise to encourage her group to help one another. Only if solutions are not forthcoming from the group, or those which do emerge are inadequate, need she intervene to give her own answers. In this way inexperienced parents can have the benefit of a variety of solutions, perhaps more detailed and more up-to-date than the solutions which a professional will have acquired during the course of her working life. Solutions given by mothers of two-year-olds may even seem more credible than the same solutions given by a professional whose children are teenagers![3] While encouraging contributions from the group, the teacher retains a responsibility to correct misstatements, and to supply balance, by pointing out that one person's experience which leads her to stress advantages or disadvantages will not necessarily either be repeated the second time round, or be true for other people. She will still be teaching, but teaching differently, and in the process gaining information which will help her to pitch the subsequent, more traditional teaching on the process of breast feeding at the right level for the particular group before her.

Brighter Teaching

Discussion periods are very helpful as a preliminary to subjects about
which the group may know little, but the teacher may know a lot. They
can also be used as an alternative to the talk, and one which is a lot
more fun for everyone. It is very difficult for a teacher to give an
interesting talk about something already taught in the same way seven
times this year, and there is a limit to new ideas for brightening up the
topic. Using the group to supply variety will make the class more
interesting for everyone. An example of this sort of approach can be
found in this extract from a class on home safety and the layette. These
are topics too often taught to little effect in late pregnancy; this
evening class for both parents was timed for early pregnancy, when
some of the shopping remained to be done. The group have just had a
tea-break; the health visitor pulls the group together and hands over to
the midwife:

Transcript 3

15.6	HV	(Your bit now — on layette) ((footstep noises))
15.7	MW	Our layette isn't (sparkling) is it
15.8	HV	No it isn't not really — it's a bit old-fashioned but still ( )
15.9	MW	Somebody's bought about ten thousand vests haven't they
15.10	UF	( ) it's her fault
15.11	HV	How many vests have you two bought
15.12	Mary	Well I've got three
15.13	Nick	63 last week — she bought
15.14	Jane	Three the first size and three in the second size I've got
15.15	Mary	( )
15.16	MW	And how many first size ones have you bought Julie
15.17	Julie	Eight
15.18	HV	*Eight*
15.19	Julie	Eight
15.20	MW	Eight tie ones — right girls three second hand vests ((2.00)) right what possessed you to buy eight
15.21	Julie	(Oh I don't know)
15.22	MW	What sort of vests have you bought
15.23	Julie	(Those that tie)
16.1	Bert	Is that what they call in*vest*ing for the future
16.2	UF	(I've got woollies) as well ((general talk))

16.3	MW	(I should er —)
16.4	Bert	Eric Morecambe's got nothing to worry about there

                       (1.0)

16.5	MW	If you're going to you know use these put them on back to front
16.6	Julie	Yes that's what nurse (**) said
16.7	MW	Otherwise they gape — see how that's gaping

        (   ) you've got it all at the back and
nothing at the front and you can always put another
new piece of tape there just inside that keeps them
together (   ) for a working minimum you
only need to have three to four first size baby vests —
because you don't need to change them (every) day
unless sicked or wet round (here)

16.8	Julie	(I'm thinking of) change them twice a day ((laughter))
16.9	MW	To get the wear out of them / / ( )
16.10	Jane	( )

she'll be changing them four times a day ((laughter))

This sounds much more fun than a little lecture on what to buy for baby. It is also more useful; the midwife suggests resale to the group as a solution to Julie's eight vests (15.20) and later on the health visitor suggests she swops with someone else who turns out to have 14 nighties. In addition, the midwife can tell Julie how to use and adapt her existing tie vests rather than telling the whole group not to buy them, advice which would come too late for her. This shows the advantages of a technique which 'pitches' advice appropriately.

The discussion is an alternative not only to the talk, but also to the film. Films can precipitate a style of teaching which might unkindly be described as 'film plus burble'. The professional turns off the projector and talks about the film, picking out bits and pieces which she wants to emphasise, or contradict as being untypical, or explain where the film was, she fears, not very clear. Intermittently she may ask the audience whether they have any questions; dazed from the combined effects of the film and the 'burble', they fail to produce any in the second or two of silence which she can tolerate, and she starts again on another tack. Silences always seem longer to the person asking for questions, or asking a clear question, than to the person desperately trying to think of a question to ask, or an answer to give. 'Film plus burble' is a common problem of beginners, since they are likely to be preoccupied with keeping going and have little attention to spare for their group's reactions. Unfortunately beginners do not always solve this problem even when they have gained experience.

The following extract is not an example of simple, beginner's 'burble' — though we have all done this in our time. It is, on the contrary, high level 'burble', an attempt to solve a number of specific, awkward problems, not to cope with beginner's nerves. Anyone using films dreads the time when the wrong film arrives. The midwife and health visitor here had wanted a film on home safety featuring very young children, suited to the situation of an antenatal class. Instead they found a film featuring older children, nine-year-olds, but still on home safety. They had wanted a film because the group they were teaching came from a poor area of the city and they thought that the emphasis from pictures and soundtrack would be better for the group than their unaided efforts. Further, the film did have a baby in it, and did feature some of the common dangers to small children — medicines, prop feeding, cookers, unguarded fires. They decided to show the film, and try to adapt it to the audience afterwards. The health visitor attempted to do this, incorporated a home safety leaflet, and lots of suggestions for home safety equipment, based on her own researches in the shops. Unfortunately, the result is, like all 'burble', long and rambling, which therefore makes it extremely difficult for people to remember specific details. A short extract gives the flavour:

Transcript 3

6.1 HV   (   ) as well make sure that toys are *good*
             toys — toys are important to children and you're better
             spending a lot of money on one — good — toy than
             cheap toys a lot of them (a lot of cheap toys are
             rubbish) cheap toys (that break) you see the bears with
             their eyes that come out it's ever so easy (kids are very
             nimble they) twist and screw and when they get to
             about 12 months — they *are* wanting to know how
             things work (they do it automatically) pull and twist
             and turn and they solve it before you know where you
             are — you saw that child in the garden shed in the film
             and what happened to one of our colleague's daughters
             — she (drank paraffin and was very badly burnt so)
             don't hesitate you know if you're worried about a
             child get them (to hospital) don't hesitate (   )
             (in the hospital) — if you practise these things now
             when you have your baby it's second nature cause it's

easier when there's only two of you —

This monologue, broken very rarely indeed, included about 30 separate safety points before the health visitor managed to stop herself talking and involve the group rather more. Monologues are addictive.

Kicking the 'burble' habit may mean *considering* giving up films as well. Considering means what it says. Films may be useful for particular purposes. The birth film is institutionalised as a feature of most ante-natal classes, and there are good reasons to support this; showing a film gives expectant parents some idea what the process looks like, and provides them with materials from which to fantasise. However, no film is ideal; the local hospital is never quite like the one on the film, obstetric practices change, women's fashions change. A number of older films do not feature fathers doing anything useful. Shots of a stretching perineum may upset some people, blood needs explaining away, procedures need explaining. All these things invite the professional showing the film to 'burble'. Before committing herself to using a film at all, she should therefore consider whether it is absolutely necessary, or whether more flexible visual aids, like slides or pictures, might not be better.

If a film must be shown, it would help to have some plan in mind to cover what to do when the projector is turned off. One safe ploy is to ask the group what they thought of it; someone may have a clear opinion. The question may need phrasing to focus on which bit they liked best or found most interesting or most relevant, or on whether, in the case of a birth film, the film showed what they had expected birth to be like. An opening like this will give some idea of the response of the group, and also act as primary prevention of 'burble'. It may also be possible then to ask the group to do some of the job of adaptation themselves. In the particular instance of the home safety film, the film referred to problems of stairs and falls; the health visitor mentions, as safety tip number 30, solutions to this:

Transcript 3

11.3	HV	((Footstep noises)) well I went round Mothercare today to find out what other things they had in safety — play pens — gates — gates you get their gates for £7.75 (but Dads if you're good) you can knock them up with a bit of wood and put two hooks so you can take it upstairs and fasten it on the upstairs bit so that
12.1		when they're upstairs they can't get downstairs and when they're downstairs they're downstairs and they

            can't *get up*stairs

12.2 Bert   The trouble is we thought of doing that (
)

12.3 HV   Have you got can you make those sort of things your-
             self

12.4 Jane   Yes

12.5 Bert   Well you can do − well you can make them − they're
             not particularly hard are they I don't think

12.6 HV   But think about lining your windows if you've decided
             on what room it's going to be the nursery − putting
             bars at the windows because those whole windows are
             big aren't they − in modern houses

12.7 UM   Mm

12.8 Jane   They swivel as well − which you have to watch (
)

12.9 HV   Yes

12.10 Jane   (   )

12.11 HV   They come out very quickly − shoot out − and they
             do − oh they love it yes they like to walk on the
             windowsills too − as a general rule − see how far they
             can walk round without (falling off) − they don't see
             danger − children (   )

12.12 Jane   I don't remember doing things like that − I probably
             did but

12.13 HV   Well I don't think − not every child did but there are
             some that are just that bit more adventurous than
             others

Bert and Jane have clearly (12.2, 12.8) started to think about
adapting their house to keep their baby safe. Bert decides, without any
encouragement visible in the transcript, to make this clear, and his
initiative is welcomed by the health visitor; she continues to make unrelated safety points (12.6) but from here onwards her utterances are
much shorter and the group, particularly Bert and Jane, make much
more of a contribution. The health visitor earlier made efforts to
encourage Mary, the only experienced parent in the group, to talk.
This was not, however, very successful, since Mary's contribution was
nearer to that of an awful warning, since she *had* prop fed her baby.
Her main suggestion of additional safety problems had more to do with
the naughtiness of the action (putting plastic toys on the fire) than the
safety risk. This sequence shows that alternatives to the monologue can

come from the intervention of inexperienced parents, when they have thought about the problem; Bert and Jane's previous planning could have been elicited earlier and used as an implicit model for other expectant parents in the group to tackle other problems raised by the film.

Teaching Through Discussion

If the teaching of some topics may be improved by more use of discussion and less of exposition, others are not suited to professional exposition at all. Family matters come into this category; social change has resulted in too much diversity in standards for professional fiat to be either acceptable or useful. Leading a discussion on such issues is a much better idea. It is, however, rather more difficult than encouraging a group to talk, in order to establish how to 'pitch' a subsequent professional exposition, or working through what to buy for baby with contributions from group members. If professional staff are uncertain about the nature of family life, it is hardly fair to ask an antenatal class to expound their views instead. It is unlikely to be useful to ask general questions, such as 'What is the nature of family life in the modern world?' Instead simpler questions can be used, phrased to lead the group to construct a picture which the leader has had in mind from the beginning.

This picture should be a representation of the 'problem', rather than the 'solution'. It is important this representation should be based on fact, not opinion. This means using accounts of individual experience from members of the group, or specially invited visitors, and using professional expertise to balance any contributions based on an experience which is not very common. In this way expectant parents can be presented with material which carries the authority of personal experience, but can be protected from assuming that what is true for others will necessarily be true for them. Similarly, solutions offered by others can be shown to be what they are — adapted to individual circumstances and not necessarily suited to everyone. A solution which involves grandmother, for example, only works for others if they have a grandmother available. Those without such a valuable standby can be encouraged to think of friends or neighbours who are experienced with babies, to whom they could turn in time of need. Indeed, they could be encouraged to cultivate such friendships before the need arises. Discussion can pose the problem clearly, aided by the teacher's ability to emphasise important points and identify a typical experience for what it is; it can also start people working towards their own solutions.

Application of this technique to family matters is sensible because no one knows the right answers on how to run a family, though professionals can identify some of the wrong ones. It can also be applied in situations where the reason for professional uncertainty is slightly different. Some teaching problems arise not because no professional answers are available, but because the detailed answers are known by other groups of professionals to which the teacher does not belong. Thus community staff preparing women for hospital delivery have problems, since their knowledge of current hospital routine cannot be a detailed and intimate one.[4] To argue for concentration of preparation for childbirth in hospital is no solution to this difficulty, since it is likely to result in fewer women attending these classes, because of transport problems. If, as seems likely, community staff must continue to prepare women for hospital, they can be helped in this task by good hospital-community contact, and by the opportunity to take their class round the delivery suite and the postnatal wards. However, they will still have some problems in explaining the social environment of the hospital. Hospital staff will, of course, know this well, but may have difficulty in seeing it from the patient's point of view, precisely because they are so familiar with the routine.

Discussion techniques may help with both problems. New parents can supply the detail on, for example, precisely how husbands staying with their wives in labour can get breakfast at the hospital, or where the coffee machine is, and what small change is needed. Community staff may lack this sort of information. New parents can also identify more readily than professionals those details which uncertain prospective patients would like to know, because they probably wondered about them too. In this field, they are experts, and their expertise is a gift to the teaching professional. She should use it. Her skills are here best deployed in teaching indirectly, by question rather than by answer. How this can be done is illustrated in the following extracts. These are taken from the last of a six session evening class for both parents. The expectant mothers, all first-timers, are in mid-pregnancy. Two sets of visiting parents, with babies of about six weeks to two months old, attended a previous course and have been invited back to talk about their experiences of birth and adjusting to family life. The session is primarily the health visitor's responsibility, with the midwife contributing on specifically midwifery topics where appropriate. Mrs A had a premature baby, and is talking about her period of 'baby blues' (introduced as 'depression' by one of the expectant fathers):

Transcript 4

6.13 Mrs A   Then of course it was building up to the day when I'd
got to come out and leave her behind anyway — which
was er — wasn't very nice but you get over that — you
know (   ) did you have a depression

6.14 Mrs B   Not really depression — I had a few weepy days but —
I think — that was tiredness more than actually being
depressed

6.15 Mrs A   Mm

6.16 Mrs B   (And also with all the visitors coming in)

6.17 Mrs A   Mm

6.18 Mrs B   (It was a bit much really, but I wasn't actually depressed)

7.1   Mrs A   I mean I was tired when she first came home
(   ) but I don't think you — appreciate the twenty four hour job ((laugh)) — getting up in
the middle of the night with your feeds and that — and
if you can't get your rest and your sleep — (it gets) you
down

7.2   Mr A   (trying to get her routine — routine
put) baby on the bottle ((laughter)) you know it

7.3   Mrs B   (Did you   )
((Lot of clinking of cups, murmurs, bangs etc))

7.4   UM   (   )

7.5   HV   Were you really

7.6   UM   (Yeh   )

7.7   Mrs B   They were there sort of — not allowing you to get into
a routine

7.8   Mrs A   (more or less have to stay
with them) (   ) (nappies or something like that — you have to sit with them) and then
you find another feed time comes round and you
haven't *done* anything and (there's everything else to
do)

7.9   Mrs B   Mm

7.10 HV   When did you feel that you'd *found* a (routine)

7.11 Mrs A   I haven't got one now ((laughter))

7.12 HV   ((2.0)) (   )

7.13 Mrs B   Not really — er — some days go marvellously and — in
between feeds I can get lots done and then other days
I seem to be feeding the whole time (and changing him

just don't do anything) — today I've had a
day like that — er — but yesterday was marvellous and
(I did loads)

7.14 HV   And you're still breast feeding aren't you
7.15 Mrs B   Yes — yes
7.16 MW   It does (   ) ((3.00))
8.1   (take a while — breast feeding is established it's just
             getting into routine it does take time)
8.2 Mr B   But these things get done — I mean — (   )
             at the end of the day (   )
             it took me five hours to (wipe) through a shirt
             ((laughter))

Note the way in which the discussion gradually shifts from 'the weeps'
to contributory factors — tiredness (6.14), visitors (6.16) and twenty-
four-hour responsibility (7.1). 'Routine', or rather the lack of it, comes
up as a sideline to twenty-four-hour responsibility, and it is the health
visitor who converts it clearly into a topic on its own by her question
at 7.10. She also points the question forward, past the period of postnatal muddle, thus establishing for the inexperienced parents that
routines do emerge. While Mrs A does not support her in this forward
look (7.11), Mrs B can to some extent (7.13). The midwife can add
professionally soothing comments about breast feeding and routine
(8.1), and Mr B is quite optimistic at the beginning of his comment,
and can joke about the problem at the end (8.2).

Despite this clear and effective professional guidance, health visitor
and midwife are unobtrusive. The health visitor only speaks four times,
and the midwife twice in this extract of 24 utterances. They are also
relaxed. There are two short pauses, of two seconds and three seconds
respectively, where the professionals wait to see if anyone else wants
to talk before they fill the gap. In particular, at 7.11/7.12, the health
visitor waits a little, giving Mrs A a chance to expand on her statement
of routine, or Mrs B a chance to comment without being asked.
Nothing happens and she says something (inaudible, 7.12) which has
the effect of persuading Mrs B to answer the question. Compare this
with the effect of speed in the health visitor's talk in Transcript 3, 6.1
(page 116) where no pause is as long as a second.

The first extract from Transcript 4 is an example of professional
guidance. The following one shows the effective way in which one of
the parents raises a new topic and makes a point which professionals
might often try to make themselves:

Transcript 4

18.12 Mr B I think one other point worth (mentioning) is that um
— on occasions — crying — and you think ooh what
you crying for — (noisy little blighter) — and then you
suddenly realise that something's wrong — that he's
covered in mess or — he's been sick and we've not
noticed it or — whatever but er — (most babies   )
they tend to cry when there's something wrong — that
you've not noticed or not done — overall you know —
as long as you feed and change them and wash them —
um — they're quite content

19.1 Mr A Well (if our kiddie's) crying it's because she tends to
want a bit of — // of attention now

19.2 Mrs A   Well naturally —
she's older than (   )

19.3 Mr A (   ) makes a mardy
cry — if (//   ) picks her up (   ) it
stops // straight away

These are the voices of parental experience speaking, used by the professionals to teach in a way that they could not improve on. Similarly,
unsolicited praise for professionals from these invited parents comes in
to great effect at the end of a discussion of conflicting advice, started
by one of the expectant mothers:

Transcript 4

21.3 UF Do you find that many people keep telling you to do
different things

21.4 UF Yeh

21.5 Mr A Yeh

21.6 UF Interfering

21.7 Mr A Yeh — I've got (   ) and you know er
— I mean they're only trying to help but —

21.8 Mrs A (   )

21.9 UF (You do your own thing don't you)

21.10 Mr A Some of their ideas may be good but some of them
says — (my) mother came in — and the wife brought
the nappies down in — you know Napisan and —
you've got to boil those — you know (you've
got to boil them every day not once a week) ((laughter
and several speaking at once)) (   ) —

that's dirty that is — so (simple   )

21.11 Mrs A It's difficult — you know — as you say I mean you've
just got to use a bit of tact and you say oh yes that's
a good idea (but er   ) I do find the midwife though a tremendous help and the health visitor
really (I thought   ) and mention it you
know if I've got any problems — just see the health
visitor and they're very good I think (
                    changed now) haven't they

21.12 Mrs B Oh yes (   ) ((laughter))

21.13 Mrs A Oh no (   )

22.1 Mrs B (   )

22.2   But I think if at the back of your mind you know
there's somebody there — you know if you *have* got a
problem ((laughter. Baby noises. Everyone speaking at
once — possibly to or about the baby))

The professionals do not need to say a word. What better advertisement could anyone want?

The Nervous Teacher

This chapter has suggested various different ways of improving response
to need in group teaching, by increasing the teacher's information on
what these needs may be, by involving members of the group in helping
one another, and by facing controversial topics in such a way as to
illustrate problems rather than give pat answers. All these strategies
have in common an emphasis on the teacher thinking seriously about
what her group may contribute to the teaching session, and how she
may help them to do this, rather than being preoccupied by her own
performance in isolation. These alternative ways of approaching group
work bear on the problem of group work nerves touched on earlier in
this chapter, and in the previous one. At its simplest, thinking about
other people's difficulties and hesitations in contributing can take a
teacher's mind off her own problems; on a more sophisticated level,
while responsibility for a 'good' session may still lie with the teacher,
recognition that others beside herself can and should contribute to the
session can relieve her of the heavy burden of pretending to be the
fount of all knowledge and wisdom.

However, it does no service to anxious beginners to pretend that their nerves will cease to trouble them if they can only be unselfish enough to concentrate on other people's problems and not on their own. This is merely to dispose of one reason for concealing nerves (that 'good' teachers aren't nervous) and to substitute another (that unselfish teachers aren't nervous). Either reason encourages those whose group teaching is a small part of their job to treat their nervousness as a shameful weakness and talk about it only with considerable caution. Myths about the ease with which everyone else handles group teaching can therefore readily persist, encouraged, of course, by the veneer of professional confidence which may be second nature to all but the trainee or the newly qualified. If no one else looks nervous, and no one talks about it, it is easy to imagine that nerves are your personal problem. This is understandable, but a mistake.

A more fruitful approach to group work nerves is to recognise that they have a function. Group teaching is a performance, not a social conversation; it is more of a performance than a clinical interview, and therefore more demanding. Some sense of excitement at the prospect of meeting a class is a form of nervous tension, and probably inseparable from a wish to do the job well. For some, perhaps, the more experienced or the more extrovert, excitement is an adequate description of the way they feel — providing certain conditions are met. They can define nerves out of existence, as some women, following what may be broadly described as the Sheila Kitzinger approach to childbirth, can define pain out of existence. For both groups this is a subjective reality; it may well also be true that both groups are a small minority. Neither approach is likely to work in the wrong conditions; both depend, in part, on a confidence which is based on adequate preparation beforehand. A teacher unsure about what she has to say, or how she intends to say it, has every reason to be nervous. Thorough preparation may or may not abolish nerves, or pain in childbirth, but it helps, and the activity involved in preparation can keep your mind off the problem to some extent. To take the analogy further, childbirth is generally a co-operative activity. Pain, or the expectation of pain, is likely to encourage a woman to look for expert help. In group teaching, a teacher should look for expert help also, from those whose expertise is differently based from her own, the members of her group. Using their knowledge of themselves and their past experience will help her, and may also free her from the fear of losing face because she does not know everything. In small group teaching, as in childbirth, no one need cope alone.

Preparation, using the help of the group, and experience will ease the

nervousness which many teachers feel before a class. There is a sense,
however, in which at least excitement, and perhaps some nervousness
are part of the process, a part of wanting to do the job well. To recognise that nervousness beforehand, and a sense of exhaustion afterwards,
are an occupational hazard for many teachers, at least makes it possible
to identify and accept a personal pattern, rather than complicate it by
a public denial of its existence. Group work nerves, then, are not a
shameful weakness; but nor are they an excuse for bad teaching. Those
who admit their nerves deserve sympathy, and, depending on the extent
to which nerves are publicly acknowledged among their professional
colleagues, may deserve respect for their courage. Once the issue is out
in the open, however, respect should be due not to what they say, but
to what they *do* about it. This means proper preparation, including an
assessment of what the group can contribute to the learning process
which the teacher is directing. This chapter has shown ways in which
teaching based on such an assessment could be developed from existing
patterns of work.

List of Symbols Used in Transcription

20.3	:	Page 20 of transcript, utterance 3
// or [[	:	Overlapping talk. Overlapping utterance positioned under overlapped utterance at point of overlap
*	:	Syllable in a name, omitted for anonymity
—	:	Pause of less than a second
(4.00)	:	4 second pause
( )	:	Something said, but transcriber cannot discern it
(heart)	:	Transcriber thinks 'heart' was said
((laughter))	:	Description, not transcription
italics	:	Indicates emphasis by volume, precision or tone
=	:	Indicates latching — one word starts immediately on conclusion of another
:	:	Indicates prolongation of syllable
?	:	Marked rising intonation
HV	:	Health visitor
MW	:	Midwife
UF	:	Female, unidentified
UM	:	Male, unidentified

This list of symbols is a grossly over-simplified version of that developed by Gail Jefferson.

Notes

1. The interpretation of 'what is happening' in these transcripts is very much specific to the sort of chapter this is, and relies in considerable measure on the discussion of the material with the midwives and health visitors concerned. It is recognised that strategy and action are not transparent in data like this. The methods used to collect this data, some problems in interpretation, and the possible benefits for improving practice by self-assessment, are outlined in Elizabeth R. Perkins and D.C. Anderson, *Self Assessment in the NHS: Techniques for Monitoring and Research* (Nafferton Books, Driffield, 1980). The use of video recordings to illuminate the problems of teaching in higher education is detailed in M.L.J. Abercrombie and P.M. Terry, 'Talking to Learn: Improving Teaching and Learning in Small Groups', Research into Higher Education Monographs (Society for Research into Higher Education, University of Surrey, 1978).

2. From the study outlined in N.J. Spencer, 'The Identification and Management of Illness by Parents of Young Children', unpublished MPhil thesis, University of Nottingham, presented 1980; quoted in D.C. Anderson, Elizabeth R. Perkins and N.J. Spencer, 'Who Knows Best in Health Education?', Occasional Paper 19 (Leverhulme Health Education Project, University of Nottingham, 1979).

3. E. Rogers and F.F. Shoemaker, *The Communication of Innovations* (Free Press, New York, 1971), discuss the superior credibility of lay sources for certain types of communication.

4. Elizabeth R. Perkins, 'Antenatal Classes in Nottinghamshire: The Pattern of Official Provision', Occasional Paper 9 (Leverhulme Health Education Project, University of Nottingham, 1978). See also Chapter 3.

7 THE POSSIBILITIES OF TEACHING IN THE HEALTH SERVICE INTERVIEW: THE PROBLEMATIC CASE OF THE CHILD HEALTH CLINIC DOCTOR

Elizabeth R. Perkins and Digby C. Anderson

Why Education?

This chapter differs from the previous six in being both more tentative and in some ways more complex. In it we have set out to look for problems with the approach used in the earlier studies of teaching on labour wards, in antenatal classes, and through clinic literature. These three settings have in common an acceptance by the practitioners concerned that teaching is an essential part of their work. In this penultimate chapter we examine both a different setting and a different professional group. We consider the possible justifications for looking at medical interviews in educational terms; the particular characteristics of medical work in child health clinics; some problems in medical interviews on which educationalists might have useful help to give; and the limitations of educational advice. In the course of this discussion we make use of empirical evidence from audio-visual recordings of child health clinic interviews. Some of our comments on teaching in the interview setting may be applicable to other professional groups; others will be specific to the medical profession, or even to particular subsections of it.

When health education by health professionals is under discussion, one frequent comment is that much health education takes place incidentally, in the course of other work;[1] or, as an important variant of this argument, that it should or could take place in this way. This 'other work' is often clinical,[2] and takes place on an individual rather than a group[3] basis. We have already seen that this approach has limitations when it is applied on the labour ward,[4] despite the established tradition of the midwife as teacher, and the advantages of certain sorts of learning to women in labour. At first sight, however, its application seems easier when it is applied to the clinical interview. Here the pressures of unpredictable work-load and possible emergency may well be less severe, or absent; professional and patient are together, probably with a certain amount of privacy, considering a problem which concerns the patient's health. Why not use the opportunity to teach?

It is this argument which is used, for example, to encourage general practitioners to become involved, or more involved, or more consciously involved,[5] in health education in their surgeries, or to urge district nurses on their rounds to practise health education, or do more of it, or to do it more consciously. The implication is that health education is part of the process already — or, that if it is not part of the process, it *ought* to be. Yet these two points of view, represented by the 'is' and the 'ought to be', are radically different. For all the settings so far considered in this book, the educational perspective[6] has been one which is part of the traditions of the professional group involved. It is therefore reasonable for an outsider to examine practice in search of educational activity, to detect problems, and to suggest alternative methods of encouraging learning. If, however, the professional group concerned is not agreed that teaching is part of the job, examining the process for educational activity is, perhaps, more problematic. For even if the group is willing to accept that they are 'doing it all the time', if 'it' has no particular importance for them, why should they be interested in doing more of it, or doing it better? They may well prefer to continue doing the things they thought they were doing originally, so that the promoter of new perspectives is left to launch his ideas into a vacuum, where not even an echo is heard.

The choice of new ways to examine particular settings or processes should not be random. If, for example, a research worker wishes to examine medical interviews for educational activity, there should be a reason for this based on what goes on in medical interviews, not merely on what goes on in the mind of the research worker.[7] One valid reason for such an examination would be that some people involved in interviews, whether professionals or patients, themselves have an interest in teaching or learning.[8] This justification would be stronger if large numbers of professionals or patients expressed this view. Another good reason would be that, even if neither patient nor professional was currently aware of this, problems with interviews could be solved if educational techniques were used. Thus one might, theoretically, appeal to evidence that patients are less likely to return with the same complaint to a professional who teaches them either how to avoid it, or how to deal with it themselves, or to evidence that compliance with medical advice is improved by more teaching by the doctor. Alternatively, one might examine the process of clinical interviewing to look for problems which an acquaintance with teaching techniques on the part of the professional would help to avoid. This second approach pre-

supposes that educationalists do have a store of wisdom which can usefully be applied[9] in the particular health setting under consideration.

Doctor-patient Interviews

Many of these reasons for taking an educational perspective on health
service work cannot be used with confidence in the case of doctor-
patient interviews.[10] As a profession, doctors are by no means agreed
that teaching is part of the job, though some doctors are enthusiastic
supporters of health education by other professional groups, like school
teachers or health visitors, or even of patient education, undertaken by
doctors. Patient complaints about lack of information from doctors are
well documented;[11] the question of what patients expect, or treat as
integral to the process of seeing the doctor, is likely to be heavily influenced by the behaviour of doctors in their previous experience, and
there is some evidence to suggest that while patients appreciate information, they do not necessarily expect it. Certainly they frequently
fail to demand it. To the extent that patient dissatisfaction with doctor-
patient interviews exists, it *may* be related to a lack of educational
activity on the part of the doctor, but there are plenty of other possible
causes, for example medical bad manners, a failure to treat patients as
individuals, or an apparent unwillingness to take the patient's problem
seriously.[12] These factors would be important whether or not the
interview was first agreed to be educational.

The arguments for improving the process through educational techniques have similar weaknesses when applied to doctor-patient interviews. Whether education by doctors can prevent patients returning
with the same problem presumably depends on the problem. In addition, doctors sometimes pass on this aspect of their work to other
professionals; the dietitian, for example, not the consultant, is responsible for teaching diabetics what food they may eat, at what times, and
in what quantities. Whether doctors still have problems in their own
contacts with patients which could be remedied by educational techniques could be detected by an examination of the interviews themselves.[13] When considering teaching techniques, however, it is worth
noting that the store of wisdom which educationalists have accumu-
lated has much to do with preplanning and group work;[14] it has less to
do with improvisation in one-to-one interviews. While there are useful
strategies which educationalists have developed for explaining, for
eliciting information and for assessing understanding of information
both given and received, these must still be adapted to suit the particular setting in which they are used — and an interview is clearly very

different from a classroom or seminar.

A justification for taking an educational perspective on medical interviews thus can depend on the doctor's and the patient's assumptions, which will be in part related to their previous experience as professional or patient, and in part governed by the problems which bring them together. These varying problems can be seen as resulting in three main types of interviews, which are unlikely to be found in their pure form in practice, but are useful for starting points for analysis. These are: the primary care interview, the screening interview, and the referral interview.[15] In the primary care interview, the patient seeks out the doctor with a problem on which he wants medical advice; usually he is, in his own definition, sick. In the screening interview he may well be summoned to attend by the health service; he may be aware of no particular problem or none that would otherwise, in his view, have merited medical attention; his decision to attend may be based on compliance with authority, or in a willingness to have his check-up and be reassured that all is well. In the referral interview the patient has made the initial effort to go for help, or to respond to a screening programme, but he has not necessarily anticipated that this would involve further sessions with a different person, concerning problems he may not have known about or which he may have defined differently. The patient's position in these different types of interview may therefore be expected to vary.

Similarly, the doctor's position may vary. A doctor conducting a primary care interview expects to see sick people, and has treatment at his disposal; his prescription pad lies ready on his desk. In a screening interview, this is not necessarily the case; the doctor's job is to check for a series of abnormalities, in the knowledge that in a proportion of cases no abnormalities will be found. Some screening services are institutionally separated from treatment, and an abnormality detected means a referral to another doctor — or another appointment in a clinic devoted to treatment. Referral interviews start, for the doctor, with some background on this particular 'case', contained in the request for referral; in the primary care interview, background knowledge, where the doctor possesses it, will be of the patient's personality and previous, possibly unrelated, complaints, rather than purely of his clinical condition. Given these different starting points for both doctor and patient in different types of interview, it is important to consider the background against which particular clinical interviews are set, and the intentions of the parties concerned, before attempting to justify an education perspective on particular interviews. Features of the practical setting,[16] including why people are there in the first place,[17] will affect both what is done, and what can be done if people want to experiment.

Child Health Clinics

Child health clinics in Britain cater for children under five and their parents, and are normally run by the Area Health Authority, though some general practitioners run child health sessions for their own patients. AHA clinics are staffed by clinical medical officers, health visitors, and clinic nurses. Broadly, clinic nurses are involved in the more routine work of the clinic, such as weighing babies, and they may, after special training, carry out immunisations under the direction of the clinical medical officer; health visitors are there to provide advice on baby care, and to carry out certain screening procedures, such as hearing tests. Clinical medical officers check that children are fit to be immunised, and may do the injections themselves. They carry out more sophisticated screening tests and are available for general consultation either on the initiative of the mother or the referral of the health visitor. Staffing organisation and the distribution of tasks vary somewhat from clinic to clinic. One crucial common factor, however, is that the child health clinic is a service for screening and advice; the doctor can only refer, not prescribe. Child health clinic interviews, therefore, may be expected to be nearest to the analytical type of the screening interview, though of course the reality may be somewhat mixed.

The role of the clinic doctor is open to considerable personal interpretation within this general framework. Mothers may come with their children to the clinic expecting advice, or even teaching; if he wished, the doctor could leave this to the health visitors as much as possible and concentrate on screening. The data used in this chapter derive from audio-visual recordings of a doctor who was interested in health education. Since at least some mothers use the clinic to help them learn about how to look after their babies, and this particular doctor was interested in helping them to learn, there is at least a minimal case for an educational perspective on these interviews. Transcripts of interviews carried out in one clinic session provide the sort of data which enable a search for problems, to see whether better educational techniques would help to solve them.

Problems — What Problems?

A justification for adopting an educational perspective on these particular interviews on the ground that it would solve problems begins to look unconvincing immediately one begins to examine the transcripts. Their overwhelming characteristic is their lack of problems of any sort. Perhaps, however, this is because the doctor has overcome the problems? It is clear that these are not aimless conversations; both mother and doctor are there for a purpose, and are working to achieve it. An examination of these interviews can help us to understand what sort of work this is. So can the doctor's own comments on his work. This chapter will use both types of evidence to illuminate the way in which 'educational' techniques may look, when transposed into a clinical interview. This is not a full analysis of what makes these interviews 'work'; it represents a partial analysis only, as a contribution to the debate about whether clinical interviews by doctors or others are, or should be, educational. The evidence presented here suggests that an educational perspective on these interviews, in this setting, by this doctor, is justifiable. There are other justifiable perspectives on these interviews. Further, all child health clinic doctors may not conduct interviews in such a way that the interviews are educational — or in such a way that the doctors' or patients' task would be made easier if they adopted educational techniques. This could be the case, but it depends at least on the way in which doctor and patient conceive of the task. More evidence, from more doctors, with or without professional unanimity about what that task is, would be required for such a judgement to be made.

Explanations

Studies which document patient dissatisfaction with health service communication[18] sometimes provoke professional reaction on these lines 'but we do communicate with patients — it's just that the patients don't understand'. This reaction, while illogical, is quite understandable when staff try to explain and feel their efforts are not appreciated. Blaming patients for their stupidity may at times be justified, but a more constructive response is to look again at the techniques of explanation[19] which are being used; for if patients do not understand, these techniques must, by definition, be inadequate for their purpose.

Explanations can be delivered from two main points of view. The professional can offer facts structured according to his own professional logic; the sort of explanation he would offer to a colleague with, it is hoped, rather simpler vocabulary and content. The alternative is to adapt the explanation to the patient's logic[20] and starting point, which involves first finding out what these are. This corresponds to the technique of 'pitching' a talk to a group.[21] In interviews this is complicated theoretically, but simplified practically, by the professional's need to find out first what the problem *is* — thus gathering information for diagnosis and gathering information to pitch an explanation may go on simultaneously.

An illustration of this process can be found in one of the recorded interviews. Mrs H has brought her baby for a six week developmental check, and the extract quoted below is preceded and followed by developmental questions, about the birth, the baby's response to visual stimuli and noise, etc. A list of symbols used in transcription can be found at the end of Chapter 6. The question at 2.8 is, in one form or another, found in all the interviews, and acts as a request for other relevant information and as an opportunity for the mother to raise issues which concern her and on which she wants the doctor's advice. Here it produces material on feeding:[22]

Transcript 4

2.8	Dr	Good ((1.00)) and really you have not had any worries about him at all since then
2.9	Mrs H	No — no — it's only feeding is a bit ((1.00)) // ( )
2.10	Dr	What's the problem with that
2.11	Mrs H	I can't seem to satisfy him
2.12	Dr	Oh ((2.00)) why have you had to increase the amount you give him or
2.13	Mrs H	No — I'm giving him — he has about five and a half ounces and then // that
2.14	Dr	Of
2.15	Mrs H	Cow and Gate
2.16	Dr	Yes
2.17	Mrs H	And then — about a couple of hours later probably give him a drink of water and he *still* only wants something else to eat
2.18	Dr	Yes — // yes
2.19	Mrs H	*You* know
2.20	Dr	— so it's really the — the fact that he doesn't go the full — three and a half to four // hours that you expect him to go
3.1	Mrs H	Yes — yes — // yeh
3.2	Dr	Yeh ((1.00)) yes — it's probably quite often that babies *don't* do that you know I mean there's no — there there there's no set

		rule to say that =
3.3	Mrs H	= oh no // I know that
3.4	Dr	That they that they they *must* go that length of time
3.5	Mrs H	No but two hours is rather early // I think for him to go — don't you think so
3.6	Dr	We:ell
3.7	Dr	I don't know really no // — perhaps not
3.8	Mrs H	No:o
3.9	Dr	No — I think — er — you see it's very difficult ((1.00)) that there is — for a start — um — as I say there's no written law to say that babies must go four hours between feeds — in fact we really don't know how long they *should* // be going — er — or how long they *expect* to go between feeds — ah — the four hour rule is really one that's been made rather arbitrarily really and and sort of — p — people have forced babies to go four hours because they they've really said I'm not going to feed him until four hours
3.10	Mrs H	Yeh
3.11	Mrs H	Yes
3.12	Dr	And you had fairly strict regimes in which people said — oh I'm not going to feed him till the // — the — and I'm absolutely going to go to the hour — and he's got to wait there and he can scream // and do — you know
3.13	Mrs H	Yeh
3.14	Mrs H	( ) I know ((laugh))
3.15	Dr	So — er — but basically I would have thought that it's sensible to — to go — onto a sort of demand feed regime in which — in which case — two hours // — er — you know — they — I think what you will in *fact* find — is that that he has certain times of the day — when he's um — when he'll do this // and oh yes ((laughing)) — and er — other times of the day when er — and other times of the day when he'll — he'll settle much more easily and // go for longer periods of time.
4.2	Mrs H	I (shall you) shan't I ((speaking to baby))

4.3	Mrs H	( )
		((to baby))
4.4	Mrs H	You know
4.5	Mrs H	You know at night time I'll probably feed him
		about — five six o'clock — and he'll sleep
		right till half past ten eleven o'clock =
4.6	Dr	= Well there you are you see =
4.7	Mrs H	= Then again in the night — he'll — sleep
		till three if I feed // him at ten he'll sleep
		till three and then again he'll wake up at six
4.8	Dr	Yeh — yeh — yeh
4.9	Dr	Yes — // yes
4.10	Mrs H	So — he'll probably // go five or six
		hours
4.11	Dr	So in fact
		he's not doing badly // is he really
4.12	Mrs H	And at night he's
		very good actually — touch // wood ((1.00))
		( ) you know
4.13	Dr	Yeh — yes —
		well during the day — well it's — it's — you're
		very fortunate that it's that way round ((laugh))
4.14	Mrs H	Yes ((laughing)) (just as I said) ((7.00))
5.1	Dr	I think what you're really describing — that a
		baby has these — different patterns of — of
		er — some t — some — they seem to have
		screaming hours really
5.2	Mrs H	Mm — mm
		((9.00))
5.3	Mrs H	((to baby)) Don't eat that sweetheart
		((baby grizzles))
		((3.00))

From 2.9 to 2.17 the doctor is helping Mrs H to make the shape of
the problem clear.[23] At 2.20 he makes a suggestion of why she thinks
there is a problem — that it is, in fact, her own expectations of babies'
feeding patterns that cause her to define her baby's behaviour as
abnormal. Commenting later on this extract, the doctor said:

Transcript 4C

23.6 Dr   = I think that's even more interesting in a sense as

> well because I think what is also happening there
> — when you think about it is that — um — I have
> also jumped a stage here — in that — er — with by
> implying that that's what you ex*pect* him to go —
> in other words that her expec*tat*ions — I'm deriving
> from this that it's *likely* that her expectations are
> that he should go four hours — now that's related
> to um — general — experience of mothers
> expecting their babies to do (
>) and that's =

He does not, however, have to rely on his experience alone; he has confirmation from the mother at 3.1 that he is right. It is also clear from Mrs H's response at 3.3 that a general statement that babies do not need to have an interval of precisely four hours between feeds is not an adequate solution to her problem. She already knows this. She follows up by saying, at 3.5, that her worry is not that he does not last *four* hours, but that he *only* lasts two. This gives the doctor a clearer definition of the problem, and a starting point for a more detailed explanation of the basis (or, rather, lack of basis) for past professional advice on feeding patterns. This explanation lasts from 3.9 to 3.14, with encouraging noises from the mother throughout. He commented, 'she is what would be regarded as an easy patient — 'cos she agrees with you all the time ((laugh))'. Her agreement, however, appears to be based on the suitability of the doctor's explanation to her case, which is well illustrated at 3.15/4.1, where he makes a tentative prediction about the variation she may find in feeding and sleeping times, and has it confirmed with enthusiasm, at 4.5, 4.7, 4.10 and 4.12. He can thus sum up at 5.1, leave pauses to check that this summary really is satisfactory, and move on to other questions.

The doctor's interest, in discussing this extract, was in the diagnostic techniques he was using, rather than the educational ones. Yet the same information can be used for both, and here *is* used for both; the doctor here establishes the mother's interpretation of the problem, and makes a guess at the pattern she is in fact experiencing. Mrs H's confirmation of his guesses, which are originally based on professional experience, both lead him gradually to a judgement on the problem as clinically trivial, and lead the mother to an understanding of why it is, in fact, nothing to worry about — and that she can, indeed, be thankful that the baby screams in the daytime, not during the night!

This sort of technique makes good use of the possibilities for education in interviews. If we compare this with letter pages in magazines, we see the difficulties which 'agony column' doctors have in trying to give helpful advice without having enough information to do so. In such cases they can only make a series of provisional statements and refer the mother to her doctor, and thus back to the interview setting, as this letter and reply published in the magazine *Parents* shows:

Is Over-feeding the Cause of my Child's Sickness?

My ten-week-old daughter had bronchitis at the age of two weeks and although she recovered after a week's treatment, she has had a lot of phlegm since then, which she brings up with a cough or after her feeds. She is very sick most of the time, and she brings back her feeds with a great deal of force. She is breast fed, and I feed her on demand. Sometimes she keeps the milk down for an hour or so, only to bring it back while she's asleep in her cot. Most of the time, however, the milk gushes back before any has had time to be digested. She weighed 7lb 7½oz at birth, and at nine weeks she was 12lb, so she is gaining weight. Do you think I could be overfeeding her?
Mrs S. Taylor,
Gwent.

It would be necessary to examine your little girl before deciding definitely whether she is merely being overfed or whether she has a problem which needs diagnosing and treating. There are two points on which you can feel very reassured. Firstly, you are breast feeding and therefore giving your child all possible protection against infection, and secondly, that in spite of vomiting, she appears to be gaining more than an average amount of weight, and must therefore be keeping a lot of milk down. The age of two weeks is very young to have bronchitis, and she certainly seems to be a baby who produces a lot of mucus. These symptoms are sometimes found in babies who have hiatus hernia. This is a slight problem at the upper end of the stomach which leads to vomiting, and which can usually be treated merely by thickening feeds and by keeping the baby in an upright position. It seems unlikely that your baby has any obstruction to the outflow of the stomach as she is gaining weight. I would suggest you try feeding her for five minutes or so less at each breast and keep her in an upright position after feeds. If this does not lead to an improvement, then you should talk the problem over with your doctor. He might feel that it is worthwhile referring her to a paediatrician, to exclude the possibility of hiatus hernia, and perhaps also to look in a little more detail at the nature of the cough you say she has. Above all, I think you should be reassured that she is gaining weight and developing so well.[24]

When the mother is actually present and can contribute her understanding of the event, explanations can be more precise, and more satisfactory to her, *if* she is encouraged to give her interpretation, and *if* this information is used. Had the doctor in Transcript 4 decided that he had dealt with the problem by 3.4, and immediately moved on to another question, he would have wasted the opportunity that interview work can give for this sort of individual explanation.

The problem raised by the mother in Transcript 4 was clinically trivial; the doctor made this provisional assessment early, by 2.20 at least. In this decision he used not only Mrs H's remarks, but also, as his later comment makes clear, his observations of mother and baby:

Transcript 4C

2.3	Dr	I would have said it was a low order complaint
		about feeding because of the way she came in and
		it didn't sort of um — it wasn't the way — what
		I'm trying to say is there are often ways — (fiercely)
		— almost as if it's your bloody fault this baby's
		not very good at feeding —

In the following extract the doctor is dealing with a problem which may be clinically significant:

Transcript 1

2.1	Dr	Any problems at all
2.2	Mrs J	— yes — you know he's sweating a lot on the head
		— just the head — on the sides — and some days
		um — it's not even warm he's sweating
2.3	Dr	Oh
2.4	Mrs J	Yeh — it — he's not — not just sweating
		normally I think it's too much — because when
		my husband was holding him like that — his
		whole sleeve was wet — // and he was still
		sweating // and sometimes when he's sleeping
		his pillow is all wet you know // all through
2.5	Dr	Yes
2.6	Dr	Yes
2.7	Dr	Mm

He asks further diagnostic questions, completes the sequence of developmental questions, and examines the baby, during which time Mrs J raises a problem with nappy rash. As she is dressing the baby again, he returns to the subject of sweating:

Transcript 1

7.3	Dr	If you just bring him across like that then you can finish him perhaps outside we'll just have a little — talk about this sweating business — you sit down there — um ((5.00)) he seems to be perfectly well at the moment — I can't find anything the matter with him he's — quite a happy baby and he's coming on nicely — um — the ((1.00)) sweating *could* be — just that he is a baby who produces a — you know who who — produces a lot of heat
7.4	Mrs J	Mm
7.5	Dr	And therefore — er tends to sweat a lot
7.6	Mrs J	Mmmh
7.7	Dr	Um ((1.00)) now ((2.00)) what I would have thought is *more* important though is if he were to er — have — sweating associated with — getting short of breath or um — you know going *really* pale and his breathing becoming fast and that sort of thing
7.8	Mrs J	Mm
7.9	Dr	But just sweating on its own I don't think means very much — so what I would — what I'm really saying is — you've got to look out for other things when this happens but if it just happens on its own
7.10	Mrs J	Mm
7.11	Dr	Then — as far as I can see — there is no reason to get er — concerned about it — OK?
8.1	Mrs J	Mm
8.2	Dr	And it may be just that you know there are some people who sweat a lot and others who don't — and — er — there are some babies who do this as well
8.3	Mrs J	Mm
8.4	Dr	who produce — er well my little boy — one of my boys — er — is soaked with — with sweat at night
8.5	Mrs J	Mm
8.6	Dr	And the other one isn't or if you — you know if he —

		if he goes to sleep in the car or something
8.7	Mrs J	Mm
8.8	Dr	He gets — it really is just — dripping off him
8.9	Mrs J	Mm
8.10	Dr	So um — I think that it must be that there's — there are some people who produce a lot of sweat and others who don't — and he's likely to be just one of those who does — sweat a lot
8.11	Mrs J	Mm
8.12	Dr	*But* — if it's associated with anything else then you must get in contact // with the doctor — OK?
8.13	Mrs J	I see — yes
8.14	Mrs J	Yes

This extract shows a different kind of expertise in explanation. After examining the baby, the doctor has decided that there is no apparent clinical problem. However, he is concerned not only to make it clear to the mother that all is well, but to help her to understand the boundaries of normal sweating. She gave him, at 2.4, a clear picture of what was happening, by its results 'because when my husband was holding him — his whole sleeve was wet'; the doctor uses a different technique, saying that sweating alone is normal, but when associated with other factors it may not be. He builds this up both by partial repetition, returning in general terms at 8.12 to the more specific points he made in 7.7, and by an illustration of normal sweating in his own son, at 8.4, 8.6 and 8.8, applying this to the baby at 8.10.

The doctor, reviewing this performance later and commenting on the sort of diagnostic questions he asked, commented:

Transcript 1C

| 13.9 | Dr | What I haven't told this mother which I think might have been (helpful with) that — with that anyway — was to say — what do *you* think's the matter with him — I mean why do *you* think he sweats — um — which is probably a way of — overcoming — a number of those hurdles — you may well get from her — er — or you might not — but you may get well (either) |
| 14.1 | | (   ) (not *right*) or she actually has some positive system to attach to it — um — |

— — — — — — — — — — — — — —

| 22.2 | Dr | Because the —er — I mean it's quite possible that a lot |

of people have talked to her about sweating beforehand
— whether they talked of it in the context of heart
disease or something — but it — certainly — in adult
patients and in a lot of — (   ) — if you
get for instance a baby with a lump — of any description — it seems to be — um — that — if you possibly
can — you've got to consider you've got to get some
way of finding out whether this mother is really
desperately worried about whether her kid's got a —
growth or not — you know a cancer or something —
and that's what seems to be — er — that seems very
frequently to — er — if you can bring that *out* —
whether it helps or not — it certainly helps you in
formulating an explanation and means of approaching
the physical sign that you either have or haven't
found — which is what I'm trying to present there —
but I've put it in very general way really there's
nothing the matter with this baby — // um

In this case he has not done, or indeed attempted to do, what he did
very successfully in the earlier case of the mother with feeding
problems — establish the mother's interpretation of the problem as a
basis from which to pitch his explanation. While the techniques he uses
for explanation are interesting and useful, they may not be successful if
she still has an unarticulated worry which is occupying part of her
attention. It is interesting that during this interview neither mother nor
doctor say why they are concerned about this particular symptom;
without a clinical background there is no way of telling from the transcript that sweating could be a symptom of congenital heart disease.
One explanation for the doctor's silence could be that he did not wish
to worry the mother, but when offered this explanation in discussion
with research workers afterwards he did not accept it:

Transcript 1C

12.7	DA	But you wouldn't have explained to the mother you were looking for heart disease because the baby was sweating would you
12.8	Dr	You wouldn't?
12.9	DA	*Would* you?
12.10	Dr	I don't know — I mean I wouldn't necessarily um — I know a lot of people who say you mention things

like that but I don't know whether that's necessarily
true — er — it's very difficult to know — you've got to
— it may just have been the way that I — that I (put
it) on that occasion.

This inexplicitness about what is the reason for doctor's initial
interest in the sweating is not, apparently, principled. It may instead
relate to the opportunity this baby presents, an unusual one in a child
health clinic, for the doctor to use his skills to search out pathology,
rather than to place the baby's development within, or outside, the
relevant range of normality. His interest in pathology does not lead him
to ignore the need to explain to the mother that there is, in fact,
nothing wrong, or to give her some idea of what would constitute
abnormal sweating. It does, however, lead him to a purely diagnostic
style of questioning which concentrates on reported symptoms, not
their significance to the mother, and a complementary doctor's explanation to which the mother contributes nothing but agreement. The
joint construction of interpretation and explanation which is a feature
of Transcript 4 is completely absent here.

It could be argued that pathology does not lend itself to educational
techniques; the doctor's knowledge, perhaps, is too esoteric. It is important, however, to note that the doctor concerned here was unaware
that he had not made his interpretation explicit, thought that he could
have done so, and thought that he should have established the mother's
interpretation. Pathology may make things more difficult for an edu-
cationally-minded doctor, but it seems open to question, and to experiment, whether they make education impossible.

Establishing an Agenda

One of the reasons for establishing patients' views of their problems is
to enable reassurance to take place. This, it has been argued, is not just
for humanitarian reasons, but because if patients are worrying about
something which has not been discussed they may not be able to understand clearly what they are being told. Studies of patients' views of
communication with doctors suggest that patients find difficulty in
raising problems;[25] doctors are familiar with, and often irritated by, the
patient who only manages to raise the 'real' problem on the way out,
after the doctor has spent time on what turns out to be a trivial presenting problem. Doctors could contribute to a solution, if they wished
to do so, by making it easier for patients to state more than one problem during the interview. Some doctors will not wish to do this, as this

extract from the Royal College of General Practitioners' publication
'The Future General Practitioner; Learning and Teaching' shows:

> The doctor may insist on focussing on certain aspects of the
> patient's problem because they are the easiest for him to handle. He
> will then refuse to allow the patient to tell him anything else, or
> refuse to hear. To obtain his greatest satisfaction the doctor usually
> wants to find a patient with a serious, acute illness that has interes-
> ting features — elicited and recognised by him with great acumen —
> and one who responds rapidly, completely and gratefully to proper
> therapy.[26]

For those who take a different approach to patient care, who prefer
to know the dimensions of the problem even if they cannot solve it, or
simply want to be sure the patient is listening to them, not wondering
about how to raise the second or third problem on their mind, a consideration of the way in which agendas for interviews are established
may be relevant to their work, as it is certainly relevant to the success
of any teaching that goes on. Teaching is ineffective if the learner is
paying no attention. In primary care interviews, the patient is at least
likely to have the chance to raise one problem at the beginning of the
interview, since in many cases the doctor can have no idea why the
patient is there. Screening or referral interviews could be expected to
be more likely to have agenda problems, since the initiative for and the
purpose of the interview derives from the health service, and the
patient may have additional matters he wants to raise.

The transcripts provide material to examine agenda-setting in a child
health clinic. Part of the work is done for the doctor before mother and
child arrive in his office; official notes have been sent asking mothers to
bring their children for developmental checks and immunisations. At
this clinic there is no appointment system, but the health visitors see
mothers when they arrive, establish why they have come, and send in
the case notes together with a brief comment on the reasons why the
mother needs to see the doctor. This may be routine, for example,
'six week check', or an individual problem 'mother worried about . . .'.
The health visitors also have the opportunity to refer mothers to the
doctor who might not have particularly wished to see him, or not for
this reason; if the health visitor cannot solve a problem, she will obviously refer, and in this series of interviews there is also an example of
a mother who came to have her child immunised, but was advised to
have his development checked as well:

Transcript 3

3.4	Dr	Yes — OK — and — they also suggest he has a routine check 'cause he hasn't had one for some time is it
3.5	Mrs L	Yes he hasn't had one — mm
3.6	Dr	For er — since he was six months?
3.7	Mrs L	((laugh)) yeh ((1.00)) // I don't think there's much wrong with him ((laughing))
3.8	Dr	Right
3.9	Dr	No I'm sure there isn't but then we might as well — now we've got him — got him here.

The health service side of the interview, therefore, has a draft agenda before the mother gets through the door. The doctor confirms this agenda with the mother, also checking the baby's name, age and sex, and then goes on to give her the opportunity to raise her side of the agenda: 'Any problems at all?' This query has a dual function, in that it can alert the doctor to developmental difficulties as well as give the mother the chance to talk about things that worry her. Thus in Transcript 1 the answer to this question, at 2.2, gives the doctor a reason to check particularly carefully for signs of heart disease. It does not always produce problems of developmental interest, although the difficulties raised may be of considerable concern to the mother; thus the feeding problem in Transcript 4 is not of clinical significance, though the doctor is willing to spend time exploring it with the mother. At the end of the discussion on feeding he reverts to standard developmental questions, and closes the sequence at 5.16:

Transcript 4

5.16	Dr	((5.00)) good — all right
5.17	Mrs H	= Can I ask you about his legs — you know every so often both his legs will just really tremble — and I // ( )
5.18	Dr	Tremble?
5.19	Mrs H	Yeh — // really — go // quiver
5.20	Dr	Like that?
5.21	Dr	Yeh — quiver — // yeh — for a very brief period
6.1	Mrs H	Yeh
6.2	Mrs H	Yeh — mm
6.3	Dr	Well that's nothing to worry about — it it — well — I I — I can — I'll show you I think I can get him to do that

if you — put him on there — take his things off and we —

At 5.16 the film shows the doctor pushing back his chair and preparing
to get up to start the next item on his agenda, the developmental
examination. As he does so, Mrs H uses this break in the sequence to
ask her question, speaking immediately after the 'all right'; she has
recognised an opportunity to raise another issue, and is using it despite
the absence of an 'any more problems' question. This time the question
is nearer to development than management, since she appears
concerned about the normality of trembling. Mrs H does not, however,
finish her account of the problem, at 5.17 or at 5.19, because of the
doctor's interruptions at 5.18, 5.20 and 5.21. His statement at 6.3,
'Well that's nothing to worry about', by itself would constitute dismis-
sal of the second problem as clinically insignificant and not worth
discussing. Instead of shutting the subject down, however, he uses it as
a bridge to the development examination, thus keeping his side of the
agenda going while allowing Mrs H to continue her subject by offering
her a demonstration as implicit reassurance that the quivering is harmless. Doctor's and mother's purposes mesh tidily, the interview proceeds
efficiently, and the mother receives no rebuke for raising irrelevant
trivia at the 'wrong' moment.

It is possible, with some latitude of interpretation, to see quivering
legs as a developmental problem for Mrs H; she is concerned about
whether this is normal, and developmental checks are intended to
establish the normality, or otherwise, of the baby. The second problem
raised by Mrs J in Transcript 1, however, is nappy rash, which may distress the baby and the mother but cannot realistically be classed as
requiring a doctor's attention. Mrs J uses a different opportunity to
talk about her particular worry, raising it during the developmental
examination itself, when mother and doctor are looking at the baby
together. During this examination the doctor murmurs quietly to the
baby from time to time, and she starts to talk, at 5.10, at the same
time as one of these murmurs:

Transcript 1

5.9 Dr   ⎡ (Are you a nice boy)
5.10 Mrs J   ⎣ I sometimes think (   ) nappies
5.11 Dr   ((5.00)) Yeh — I think that's associated with his er —
                with when he gets wet from his water — from his —
                when he — when he wets his — nappies
5.12 Mrs J   Mm

5.13 Dr	And erm — it burns the skin very slightly round there
5.14 Mrs J	What shall I put ( )
5.15 Dr	Well you really need — it it needs only — to have something like — do you use zinc and castor oil — or anything // what do you usually put on
5.16 Mrs J	No — I — just use Drapolene
5.17 Dr	Yeh ((1.00)) well ((1.00)) it seems to depend very much on the — you know Drapolene works for some babies and — and perhaps doesn't for others
5.18 Mrs J	Mm
6.5 Dr	So there's no sort of er — definite — cream to give just — when you *do* put cream on ensure that you put quite a thick layer on // that's really what ( ) — there are some which are supposed to heal it up but basically the thing to do is to protect it in the first place
6.6 Mrs J	Mm — yes

The mother's comment is partly inaudible because two people are talking at once, and is somewhat tentatively phrased: 'I sometimes think'. Had the doctor wished to do so, he could have ignored the mother and continued to talk to the baby, relying on his professional prestige to maintain his control of the interview. Had he done so, he would have been acting in line with the pattern described by the Royal College of General Practitioners; he could have argued that he was there to do developmental checks, not to give advice on nappy rash. In fact he deals with the problem, establishing what the mother is doing about it currently, and suggesting extensions to her existing practice rather than condemning that practice outright.

An open agenda may have a lot to do with the existence of particular points of transition, like the shift to a physical examination, or a joint focus, like mother's and doctor's attention to the baby on the couch. Here new problems could be raised, in the same way that a transition point from one teacher to another in group work may provide a chance for questions.[27] But the use of these opportunities to raise new problems, if further problems do exist, will depend in part on the patient's estimate of the doctor's willingness to tolerate them, based on experience either of this doctor or of other doctors' behaviour in the past. If the description by the Royal College of General Practitioners is reflected in reality, patients may well expect doctors to be unsympathetic to open agendas and multi-problem interviews, and subside very quickly when their second or third questions are dismissed.

The Limitations of Problem Hunting

It was argued at the beginning of this chapter that there was a case for investigating these child health clinic interviews from an educational perspective, because mothers could reasonably be hoping to learn something at the clinic, because this doctor was interested in health education, and because it could be that there are problems in these interviews which could be eased by advice from educationalists. It has been seen that there are few problems in these interviews, and while the doctor's practice is not perfect in educational terms, as, indeed, no teacher's practice ever is, he needs no educationalist to tell him what is wrong. This doctor is doing nicely without advice from outsiders. This could be, of course, because he is a good natural teacher. It could be, alternatively, that the skills he is using are those of interaction, rather than specifically of education; his commentary on his activities focuses on different facets of his work from those a teacher would select. Thus his comments on Transcript 4 are concerned with establishing the nature of the problem, rather than with working up the explanation; yet both are possible interpretations of the evidence, and, indeed, both go together. It is in this sense that it can be argued that doctors, or, perhaps, good doctors, are 'doing health education already'. For those with an interest in this aspect of their work, who also feel that they could use some help to do it better, educationalists have something to offer, though they may do better to offer it through analysis of doctors' work than directly from teacher to doctor.[28] Advice from teachers cannot easily be assimilated into clinical interviews, since too much adaptation of teaching wisdom to medical practice needs to be done first.

   An alternative source of help from educationalists to doctors might come through experiment with visual aids. These might help to ensure that both parties were talking about roughly the same thing, as for example, on the question of pallor, in Transcript 1, or in illustrating what to look for in case of further trouble. A variant of visual aids is already available in the form of booklets and leaflets; their limitations have already been discussed in Chapter 4. Good clinic booklets might also help with the problem of retention — if the doctor gives a lot of information, how much will the mother remember? Again, leaflets or visual aids need to be appropriate to the persistent problems which do arise; it is, of course, unrealistic to hope for a booklet to suit every problem, but material written by those ignorant of the workings of child health clinics is unlikely to be of much real help.

Moreover, it is not merely a question of adaptation of either sort of advice to the interview format. Interviews are concerned with other things than teaching. Here the doctor's official concern is with developmental checks; most of the extracts featured here are his responses to problems offered by mothers, and the connection with development may be obscure or non-existent. The rest of the work has also to be done, and done against pressure of time, which, while it is not, perhaps, as serious as that on the labour ward, is still a factor which cannot readily be ignored. A long queue in the waiting room affects mothers, and through them, if in no other way, the doctor and the interview.

Teaching tips will not improve doctors who are not interested in teaching. Nor will they improve doctors whose basic medical knowledge is defective. The training of clinical medical officers for this specific post is either scanty or non-existent; the Court Report[29] recommended that this should be remedied. If it is agreed that their role should involve some educational work with mothers during interviews, examinations of practice of the type conducted in this chapter might be helpful to them. But unless their paediatric knowledge is sound, educational expertise would be wasted; indeed, it might even be harmful, since mothers would learn wrong information more easily!

There are other problems in clinical interviews which are not amenable to educational advice. Teachers have similar problems to doctors in that health education in school relates to a home situation of which teachers may have little or no knowledge, as doctors may have little knowledge of their patient's home. Similarly, health education in school or surgery tends to have implications for other members of the family who are not present, often not consulted, and may not have any enthusiasm for the change required. Both teachers and doctors have home visiting open to them as an aid to solving this problem; neither group uses it very much. Education has, at present, few tried and tested solutions to offer; indeed, schools may adopt the same expedient as doctors and pass the problem to the health visitor!

Finally, there is another kind of problem with doctor-patient interviews which is not really the doctor's problem at all, but the patient's, and there is a limit to what the doctor can do about it even if he wishes to do so. This is the problem of lack of patient self-assertion. The patients who forget problems as they get through the surgery door, or do not have the courage to raise all the ones they do remember, will undoubtedly find things easier with a sympathetic doctor who believes in keeping a reasonably open agenda. But sympathetic doctors cannot help if patients do not take their share of the responsibility for seeing that the interview works to their satisfaction. We have seen in these interviews that the mothers do not sit passively and wait for the doctor to prise problems out of them. Helping patients to assert themselves, either by rehearsal of their wishes before the interview or by suggesting that they make notes of what they want to ask before they arrive, could be a useful part of patient education in the use of the health services.[30] Educationalists might, indeed, be more usefully employed in this task than in trying to improve the teaching techniques of doctors who do not believe they are in the teaching business anyway. There are limitations to the educator's role even here, in the same way that there are limitations to their role with doctors. To what extent is assertiveness training to do with education? To what extent can people prepare the questions they will want to ask the doctor about their treatment, when they do not know beforehand what that will be? In interviews, improvisation is inevitable, and preparation thus has limits.

This chapter has shown the limits of more than preparation. It has argued that an educational perspective is not always justified; that one cannot always find problems amenable to educational solutions; and that educationalists may not have very much to offer in particular situations, even if problems which look educational can be found. These conclusions come from an examination of a particular type of doctor-patient interview, in a reasonably favourable setting for educational work. They may well apply elsewhere with greater force: to work in referral interviews by hospital doctors; to work on wards by nursing staff whose concern is care, and whose understanding of the educational component of care is perhaps somewhat more nebulous than that of midwives. All these clinical settings *may* show that education is (or should be) being carried out already. Until an examination is made both of the practical setting and of practitioners' understanding of what they are doing, it would be wise to maintain an open mind about the contribution which educational advice can make.

Notes

1. This argument is the basis for the Health Education Council's promotion of Certificate courses in health education. See also D.C. Anderson, 'Talking with Patients about their Diet', and Elizabeth R. Perkins, 'Antenatal Care and Postnatal

Nursing: Aspects of the Role of the Midwife in Health Education' both in D.C. Anderson (ed.), *Health Education in Practice* (Croom Helm, London, 1979).

2. For example, doctors' consultations with patients, midwives' and nurses' care for patients on hospital wards, and physiotherapists' rehabilitation work.

3. Unlike the organised antenatal classes discussed in Chapters 3, 5 and 6.

4. See Chapter 2.

5. The Health Education Council runs courses for general practitioners to encourage them to increase their involvement in health education during their normal work. This argument is also used in the unpublished study group report of the Royal College of General Practitioners in 1976, 'The Education of Patients and Public by General Practitioners in the Seventies'. P. Byrne and B. Long, *Doctors Talking to Patients* (HMSO, London, 1976), is relevant for a more general consideration of better communication in general practice.

6. Education is here used in the sense of teaching techniques, not as an omnibus word to cover all forms of communication.

7. D.C. Anderson, 'Abstractive and Observational Methods of Educational Evaluation in a Dietetic Clinic', paper read at the 10th International Conference of Health Education (London, September 1979).

8. As in the attention to the 'actor's definition of the situation' shown in symbolic interactionist and phenomenological sociology: D.L. Weider, *Language and Social Reality* (Mouton, The Hague, 1974); A. Schutz, 'On Phenomenology and Social Relations', in H.R. Wagner (ed.), *Selected Writings* (Chicago Press, Chicago, 1971); H.S. Becker, *Sociological Work: Method and Substance* (Allen Lane, London, 1971); A.V. Cicourel, *Method and Measurement in Sociology* (Free Press, New York, 1964); D. Phillips, *Knowledge from What?* (Rand McNally, Chicago, 1971).

9. D.C. Anderson casts doubt on this in 'Systematic and Modest Schemes for Health Education in Schools' in D.C. Anderson (ed.), *The Ignorance of Social Intervention* (Croom Helm, London, 1980).

10. There is, of course, a substantial literature on doctor-patient interaction (for example, Byrne and Long, *Doctors Talking to Patients*, and the studies in M. Wadsworth and D. Robinson (eds.), *Studies in Everyday Medical Life* (Martin Robertson, London, 1976)), but much of this does not address technical factors (W.W. Sharrock, 'Portraying the Professional Relationship' in Anderson (ed.), *Health Education in Practice*), and is neither educational nor practical (D.C. Anderson, 'The Practical Implementation of a Health Education Programme' in Anderson (ed.), *Health Education in Practice*).

11. For reviews of the literature, see Debra L. Roter, 'Patient Participation in the Patient-provider Interaction: The Effects of Patient Question Asking on the Quality of Interaction, Satisfaction and Compliance', *Health Education Monographs* (Winter, 1977), p. 281, and J.M. Clark and L. Hockey, *Research for Nursing: A Guide for the Enquiring Nurse* (HM & M, Aylesbury, 1979).

12. As shown in Elizabeth R. Perkins (ed.), 'Survey of New Mothers in Sutton-in-Ashfield', mimeo (Leverhulme Health Education Project, University of Nottingham, 1976).

13. This is an approach based on practice as outlined in Anderson (ed.), *Health Education in Practice*.

14. D.C. Anderson, *Evaluation by Classroom Experience* (Nafferton Books, Driffield, 1979).

15. Material which could be used to show the variations in different medical interviews, is included in M. Bloor, 'Professional Autonomy and Client Exclusion: A Study in ENT Clinics' in Wadsworth and Robinson (eds.), *Studies in Everyday Medical Life*, where the varying use of information based on referrals is discussed; Byrne and Long, *Doctors Talking to Patients*, considers the general practice setting.

16. Including the duration of the interview, the arrangement of furniture, the personalities, and personal histories of the people involved, their relative social status (real and perceived) and linguistic competence.

17. M. Wadsworth, 'Studies in Doctor-patient Communication' in Wadsworth and Robinson (eds.), *Studies in Everyday Medical Life*, discusses expectations of doctor and patient in more general terms.

18. See note 11.

19. 'Explanation' here refers to the intention of the paediatrician, not a particular technique; it is thus used to cover instruction, narrative or any other methods used with the *intention* of explaining.

20. See note 8.

21. Discussed in Chapter 6.

22. For the methods used to collect this data, see Elizabeth R. Perkins and D.C. Anderson, *Self Assessment in the NHS: Techniques for Monitoring and Research* (Nafferton Books, Driffield, 1980).

23. Our interpretation of 'what is happening' in these films and tapes is very much specific to the sort of chapter this is, and relies in considerable measure on discussion of the material with the doctor involved. We recognise (and indeed have ourselves argued elsewhere) that strategy and action are not transparent in data like this: Perkins and Anderson, *Self Assessment in the NHS: Techniques for Monitoring and Research*.

24. *Parents* (August 1978), pp. 9-10.

25. For example, Barbara M. Korsch, Ethel M. Gozzi and Veda Francis, 'Gaps in Doctor-patient Communication', *Pediatrics*, vol. 42, no. 5 (November 1968), pp. 855-71, using a sample of 800 mothers, found that only 24 per cent of main worries were specifically mentioned to doctors during consultations.

26. Royal College of General Practitioners, 'The Future General Practitioner: Learning and Teaching' (RCGP, London, 1972).

27. See Chapter 6.

28. N.J. Spencer and Elizabeth R. Perkins, *Evaluating Communication with Patients: Self Assessment Techniques for Doctors* (Nafferton Books, Driffield, 1980).

29. Report of the Committee on Child Health Services, *Fit for the Future* (HMSO, London, 1976).

30. See for example, Open University, *The First Years of Life* (1977), *Health Choices* (1980); also Debra L. Roter, 'Patient Participation in the Patient-provider Interaction: The Effects of Patient Question Asking on the Quality of Interaction, Satisfaction and Compliance'.

8 PLANNING FOR PROGRESS IN PATIENT EDUCATION

Tradition and Content

Professional groups concerned with the health of mothers and babies have traditionally been concerned with teaching as well as with caring and curing. Teaching is part of the job because it is clear that the understanding co-operation of parents, and action based on understanding by parents, is very important in achieving the aims of both professionals and parents — healthy mothers, and healthy children. Yet, as the studies in this book show, professional traditions and professional goodwill are not enough to ensure that patient education offered by professionals will meet patients' needs. This mismatch between intentions and practice requires explanation.

In part problems arise precisely *because* the professionals concerned have a tradition of teaching parents. If patient education was a new idea in midwifery, or health visiting, or child health, much time might be spent in thinking about what patients should be taught, and when. Asking patients for their views could reasonably be expected to be part of this process. Since teaching is a traditional activity, however, it is easy to assume that the content and timing of teaching can also be left to tradition, though perhaps methods of teaching might need revision to take account of the competition of television, for example; thus the demand for good films.

Unfortunately, tradition is not a reliable guide either to content or to timing. It is fallible for two main reasons: the rapid changes in obstetrics, paediatrics and society, and the variability of individual need. Changes in obstetric practice affect both women's expectations of labour, discussed in Chapter 3, and their need for information during labour, discussed in Chapter 2. Research in paediatrics has resulted in changes in approved child-rearing practice, and these changes are likely to continue to occur; the implications of professional controversy for parent education are discussed in Chapter 4, in the context of written advice to parents, but controversy is obviously a problem for those practitioners who teach individuals or groups directly, as well as for those who design educational literature. The effects of social change, in the increased mobility of young couples and young families, can make parents more dependent on professional advice, and yet the increased

assertiveness of consumer groups, and the increased knowledge of
alternative styles of living and of rearing children, provides parents with
precedents to query, criticise or reject professional advice. The tension
between an increased dependence on professionals, and an increasing
willingness to criticise them, may even exist in the same person. In this
minefield, professional traditions, stemming from the days when
approved practice for parents and professionals changed at a more
leisurely speed, provide no adequate guide to what parents need to
know, although they will continue to give practitioners both inspiration
and valuable clues.

Institutions and Timing

The effects of social and professional change do not only mean that professional traditions should no longer govern content in parent education.
They also call into question the institutional arrangements which the
health service has made to try to meet patients' needs. Clinics and
classes arranged at times which suit the service but not the patients
could readily result in patients not attending; in these circumstances it
is obvious that they are ineffective as a means of arranging patient
education. Thus, for example, antenatal classes which welcome fathers,
but take place in the daytime only[1] are unlikely to have much success
in educating fathers, at least in areas where many men work normal
office hours. Such anomalies may be comparatively easy to spot. A
more difficult problem to identify comes from gradual social change;
clinics and classes may continue to attract customers, but attract fewer
people, or different people from the groups for which the class or clinic
was designed originally, or attract the same people at a different stage
in their parental development. Because the changes are slow, it is easy
for experienced practitioners to continue to do what they have always
done, and not to notice that it may no longer be appropriate. One
particular example of this problem has been discussed in Chapter 5; a
proportion of topics taught in antenatal classes are not particularly
appropriate to women in late pregnancy, although they could be of
considerable value to the same women at an earlier or later stage. The
inclusion in the programme of topics appropriate to earlier pregnancy
can most readily be explained by their survival from the days when
pregnant women would not generally go out to work, even in early
pregnancy. They could thus attend classes early, whereas today most
women pregnant for the first time continue to work until they are 28

weeks pregnant, and attend classes only after this stage. Changing social patterns can thus make the timing of teaching no longer appropriate to patients' needs, although perhaps once they were entirely suitable. Similar arguments can be applied to the length of antenatal courses[2] and to the arrangements for antenatal care[3] and child health clinics.[4]

In some cases the problem of inappropriate timing can be solved by changing the institutional arrangements. Holding some sessions of an antenatal course in the evenings, for example, to cover topics appropriate to early pregnancy, or where fathers' involvement is particularly important, is not a radical new idea, but one which has already been tried by many individual antenatal class teachers. In other cases this is more difficult; in Chapter 2 it was argued that some teaching on labour could only be given to a woman during her labour, because it could not be known beforehand how her labour would develop and thus what information she would need. Yet it was also argued that the labour ward setting makes good teaching extremely difficult, and that the problems of teaching on the labour ward could not be entirely solved within the present situation. Similarly, it has been argued elsewhere[5] that while it may be possible to organise antenatal clinics to meet women's needs for information on their physical condition and on self-care, it seems improbable that clinics can also be organised so that all, or even most, women feel free to discuss their emotional problems there. While some improvements are possible in these settings, the effects of professional, rather than social, changes make it very difficult to see how appropriate teaching can be offered, at the appropriate time, i.e. during labour or during clinic care, to all women involved, without a radical reorganisation of the service. It is no part of the brief of this book to argue for such a reorganisation; instead it is argued that professionals and consumers should be realistic about what can and cannot be achieved by piecemeal reform within the existing system. Some failures to offer teaching at the right time can be remedied without major upheaval; some cannot.

The Variability of Individual Need

Professional traditions have never been able to provide more than a general outline of what patients should be taught. A modification of these traditions to take account of professional and social change can produce an improved outline, but not a final blueprint which will apply to all patients. There remains the problem of adapting to individual need. Solutions to this problem require teaching methods which involve patients in expressing their needs, and in taking an active part in their own learning. Teaching methods are discussed in detail in Chapters 5-7 in the contexts of group and individual teaching. The material used in Chapters 6 and 7, drawn from transcripts of group teaching sessions and child health clinic interviews, suggests that increasing patient involvement in the learning process is not a particularly radical thing to suggest. Some practitioners are doing this already; others could do so, without major disruption of their existing teaching styles. Development, rather than revolution, is suggested.

However, it is important to be clear about the implications of this 'development', for to some professionals it may indeed mean revolution. Finding out what patients know, or think, or feel, before starting to teach involves the health service teacher in relinquishing some professional control for part of the encounter, while patients offer personal information. This could be threatening to the teacher, since it runs counter to one received health service position: that professionals know and patients do not. It is an unfamiliar position for staff who have used their own professional traditions, or doctor's orders,[6] as a framework within which need may be defined. But educational need cannot be defined entirely in terms of the medical demands of the condition, even if these demands are adapted to those individual characteristics which can be recorded on a chart, like marital status, obstetric history, or weight. Educational need must be related also to what goes on inside the patient's head, and the only person who has access to that is the patient.

Planning Parent Education — A Two Stage Model

The problems revealed by small scale studies of parent education do not suggest that the process can safely be left to professional traditions and individual initiative. Traditions are valuable as foundations to build on, but are misleading as blueprints for a whole structure. Individual initiative is invaluable in experimental work; some individuals, however, show no initiative at all, and rely entirely on tradition. Where parents are passed from one professional to another, and offered different types of teaching on each occasion, they may finish their series of contacts confused on some points and uninformed on others, and are unlikely to feel more confident as a result.[7] The assumption that teaching is part of the job, and need not, therefore, be organised, can lead to some women being taught how to bath a baby three times in three different ways, while remaining hopelessly confused about the role of the health visitor. 'Everybody's business' can become nobody's business. But while planning and precision are valuable in education, an excess of planning and precision, at the wrong level, may make for worse practice, not for better. Management planning of group teaching, for example, where the content of each session is precisely prescribed, reduces the scope of the individual practitioner to assess individual need and teach accordingly.

So where does this leave us? Is it a choice between the strait-jacket of management planning, producing either unresponsive teaching or covert revolt among infuriated staff, and the risk of chaos as each professional interprets her teaching role as she sees fit and to the extent that she finds time? Forced choices are usually false ones, and so is this. There is a third, more demanding, but ultimately more satisfactory, course of action. Management's immediate task, I would argue, is not, at first, to plan — but to think, and to encourage their staff to think. Thought should be applied both to what information could reasonably be expected to be of use to a patient *at a particular time*, and to the nature of the setting in which such information might be given. Thinking about how to match possible needs with possible settings is easier if there is information available on what some men and women say they need, on how many people of what type attend particular settings, or read particular literature, or on the social characteristics of particular settings. Managers could consider trying to collect local information to help them and their staff,[8] as well as making use of others' research.[9]

So far this process is a professional one, with professionals only guessing at need. There is nothing wrong with this, providing the guesses are educated, not blind guesses, and that they are treated as provisional ones, to be capable of revision in the light of new inform-ation based on area studies, or new information for particular individuals. After thinking about the nature of professional work settings, and about what individual patients may need, managers and staff may see more clearly what should *not* be done. Certain inform-ation needs to be given early or not at all — for example, if smoking in pregnancy should be discontinued before a particular gestational stage to be of any benefit to the foetus,[10] it is useless and unkind to lecture women on their bad habits in late pregnancy. Other information has high priority at certain stages, but not at others; appropriate diet is an important topic, but there are others more important to teach to women who are in late pregnancy. Some topics may need a relaxed unhurried setting, or a professional well known to the patients. One example which illustrates well the sort of problems related to settings in which teaching may be attempted is the topic of lovemaking in pregnancy. The Open University Course *The First Years of Life*, a non-academic course aimed at expectant parents and parents of children under two years of age, provides material based on the assumption by the authors of the course that expectant parents would be helped by information about the safety of intercourse in pregnancy, and about possible solutions to practical problems, such as the size of the 'bulge'. If health service staff were to take this assessment of need seriously, what could they do about it? The first type of information could, perhaps, be given in a busy, anonymous, semi-public hospital antenatal clinic; it is difficult to see how the second type could be given in the same surroundings. Such information would have to be given in another way — through leaflets, or possibly during classes or home visits.

After a period of thought it may become possible to assign some topics to some settings, rule out certain combinations of topic and setting, and to consider the benefits, or drawbacks, of repetition of topics in different settings. Repetition of topics may help people to remember; in other cases, it may cause confusion. It certainly does involve more staff time. It could, for instance, be decided that community midwives should teach baby bathing to all mothers discharged after 48 hours in hospital, and that the hospital staff will not attempt to do so. A provisional framework for parent education can thus be constructed. It should not attempt to assign every conceivable topic to a setting, but only to set out those things which must be done at a certain time and in certain settings, because otherwise they are unlikely to be of benefit or even possible. This provisional framework should be written down, labelled as provisional, and circulated to all staff concerned.

At this point the focus of planning shifts from the comparatively large scale to the small scale, and from the professional community to the interaction between patient and professional. It is here that the professionals' guesses about what patients could reasonably be expected to need must be tested against individual reality. It is here that the professional needs suitable techniques to assess individual need, and to meet it where possible. Many health service professionals are more expert at doing this in a one-to-one setting than they are within a group, and here again, management may be able to help them to improve their skills. In this stage of the process management should be encouraging local initiative, to identify and to find ways of meeting local and individual need. Ideas can usefully be shared; general findings may be fed into the provisional framework, to add to it or to modify it. But the model is and remains two stage. The provisional framework should never cease to be provisional; it is general, and its conclusions will be affected by changes in the facts about places for teaching and assumptions about patient need on which it is based. It should never, therefore, attain the status of a final solution. Patient education involves learning from patients as well as teaching them. When it is working properly, it should act like a self-administered stimulant, rather than a prescribed tranquilliser.

Training for Patient Education

The argument for a two-stage planning process is based on a belief that the individual practitioner must be left enough scope to respond to each patient, or each family, or each group in such a way as to encourage the expression of particular needs, problems, beliefs, fears, or prior knowledge, and to encourage active learning on that basis. Staff should therefore be equipped with skills to make the best use of this freedom. Some are good natural teachers, or can readily build teaching skills on an instinctive sensitivity to individual need. Such professionals need little help from either basic or in-service training, except perhaps the confidence to follow their own judgement. They are the natural experimenters, whose managers should cherish and foster their initiative. However, most people can use some help. There are several levels at which this help could be provided; whether these levels correspond to basic or in-service training will, of course, depend on the training patterns of particular professional groups. Some would argue that the first level consists of visual aids: good films, or good leaflets. Area Health Education Units which supply visual aids to health service staff are under pressure to provide more and better aids. However, the limitations on patient education through leaflets and films are not only caused by the deficiencies of the available range, considerable though these may be. Leaflets and films cannot answer questions; they are in general poor methods for encouraging active learning. If they are to be used as teaching *aids*, not substitutes for health service staff, those who are to use them will need some basic teaching skills.

Specific teaching techniques, for example 'pitching' a talk to a group, or tailoring an explanation to an individual case, have been discussed in detail in Chapters 6 and 7. The widespread problems of

communication between health service staff and patients[11] suggest that
staff should be encouraged to check frequently on whether explanations have, in fact, been understood. They may also need to learn
techniques of checking which can be put into practice without making
patients feel stupid if they have not understood. These skills can be
taught. They can also be caught. There is some evidence that teachers
teach by the method by which they were last taught.[12] Student nurses,
midwives, health visitors, physiotherapists and doctors are likely to use
their tutors as models when they themselves are in a position to teach.
If student nurses, for example, are subjected to shaming as a means of
urging them to do better,[13] it would not be surprising if they either
used shaming techniques themselves with patients,[14] or never checked
whether patients had understood because they did not wish to shame
the patients by revealing their ignorance.[15]

Basic training courses may have little time available to provide
explicit guidance on teaching patients. Whether or not this is the case
with any particular professional group, tutors have the opportunity to
lay the foundations for good teaching in the future by their students.
They can teach by example, in their own attitude to informal
evaluation, or to student participation and the relevance of previous
student experience; in the importance they attach to their own ability
to know all the answers, as opposed to being able to look up information; in the way in which they handle noncomprehension, or mistakes.
This teaching by example is going on all the time, whether tutors plan
for it or not. In their own practice they will contribute much to
students' views of what it means to teach and to learn within the health
service.

More generally still, in basic training, students develop a way of
living with work which can be extremely demanding emotionally.
Isabel Menzies has argued that the student nurse is encouraged to
cultivate a professional impersonality and insensitivity to individual
patients.[16] This is a poor foundation for good teaching practice, with its
demands for sensitivity to individual needs, which may not be clearly
expressed. Nurse training is not only relevant to nurses; many midwives,
and all health visitors are trained as nurses before they train as midwives
or health visitors. Those who experienced training as Isabel Menzies
describes it, and who wish to develop their teaching skills, may have
some unlearning to do before they are able to respond fully to their
patients' educational needs. Those responsible for basic training clearly
have a role to play in helping students to cope with distressing
situations without blunting their sensitivities to the extent that they

cannot detect, and respond, to individual patient needs; in the mean-
time, trained staff may be helped either by organised in-service
programmes, or by more open relationships between health service
staff,[17] or by a combination of both. Good teaching involves relationships; it can therefore involve both risk and strain. This is not a burden
which individual staff should have to carry alone.

Assessing Patient Education

The reader who has reached this point in the discussion will be under
no illusion that patient education is a simple activity. If thought,
planning and emotional energy is to be expended on it, it seems
desirable that all this effort should result in definite achievements.
Evaluation of the health education of patients, however, is a lot easier
to demand than it is to achieve.[18] To start with, patient education can
be justified in several different ways. There is the argument from
prevention, in that some illness could be prevented if potential sufferers
understood the risks and acted accordingly. There is the argument from
cure, where cure is slow or even incomplete or absent without the
understanding co-operation of the patient. There is the argument from
professional efficiency, in that informed patients may be easier to deal
with. In varying forms these arguments can be found within the
professional traditions of teaching as part of the job. All point to
outcomes where the patient should not only understand, but also be
motivated to act in a particular way. To these arguments we may add
the moral case for patient education, that patients have a right to know
what risks they run, or alternatively what may befall them at the hands
of the caring professions. This case includes no specific requirement for
patient action, though it may be linked to a case supporting the
patients' right to make their own decisions, and thus their need for the
best possible information on which to base these decisions.[19]
    It can be seen that these arguments imply two different types of
judgement about success, failure, or more generally, standards in
patient education. Supporters of the first three arguments will be
inclined to measure success by what patients do, or do not do. For
example, such a health service teacher may wish to know whether a
patient has stopped smoking, whether she has done her postnatal
exercises, or whether she is now sterilising feeding bottles in the
approved manner. If the answer is no, then the programme has failed.
Teaching which is based on the final two arguments is likely to lead to

assessments of success measured by what patients say. If the patients say that they are well informed, that they have benefited by the teaching, or that it helped them to make decisions, then this is success. If they continue to feel ill-informed despite an educational programme, that programme is a failure, no matter how hard the staff have tried. In practice, programmes may be started for a mixture of reasons, and the criteria for judging success and failure will therefore also be mixed.

Blame for the failure of a programme may be allotted in four main ways. Probably the natural reaction for those involved is to blame the patients, at least at first, and to decide that these people must be too stupid to learn. For those outside the service, the instinctive reaction may be to blame the staff, labelling them as insensitive, prejudiced, or unable to speak plain English. Neither reaction is likely to be more than a very partial truth. A few patients may require more individual attention to help them to learn than the staff can realistically be expected to give; a few of the staff may have unfortunate personalities which make it difficult for anyone to learn from them. A more helpful place to concentrate attention is on the teaching programme itself, whether this is clearly defined, as in a series of group teaching sessions, or part of a clinical setting and therefore, in one sense, informal. If significant proportions of people do not attend teaching sessions, do not understand what they are told in clinics, or do not act on the advice they are given, then the fault may be in the design of the programme and the methods used within it. If little opportunity is given for activity on the part of the learner, or for the teachers to understand the learner's point of view before attempting to extend it to include new information or ideas, then it is likely that the programme will display educational faults and will fail for educational reasons. A third reaction to the partial or complete failure of a programme, therefore, is to reconsider what is being offered in relation to the learners' needs. Is it being presented at a time when people are receptive? Is it arranged to provide the opportunity for teachers to find out about patients' existing views and knowledge, and for patients to take an active part in their own learning? Does it take place in a suitable setting? Early failures can thus lead to improved standards.

However, educational programmes may fail for non-educational reasons. Behaviour change relies on more than information; it may be motivation that is absent. Not everyone wants to be informed about risks, or medical care. This may not be a simple matter of lack of interest; it can be traced also to external circumstances. The woman who smokes during her pregnancy, for example, may not do so because she is unaware of the risks, or because she is irresponsible. She may continue to smoke because the effects on her family of her attempts to give up cigarettes are, in her judgement, worse than the risks to her baby.[20] It may be that better educational programmes could help her to find a less harmful solution to stress than cigarettes; this would certainly be worth trying.[21] But there is no guarantee that this solution would work for everyone. Similarly, the woman who is advised to rest in late pregnancy may not do so because she has a demanding toddler. The simplest solution to her problem is not better education, but help with the toddler. Education has limitations and it is unrealistic to imply that if standards of teaching were high enough, all patients would be well informed and would change their medically inadvisable behaviour.

Beyond Parent Education

This book has concerned itself with parent education in health service settings; with parents as patients. As the title of this chapter has suggested, lessons from studies of parent education may also be relevant to educational work with patients who are not in contact with the health service in the capacity of parents or prospective parents. The advantage of studying patient education in relation to the maternity and child health services is that the teaching tradition is both explicit and long-standing. There are, however, special features of parent education in the health service which do not necessarily apply to patient education in general. For example, there is a conceptual clash inherent in the term 'patient education'. Patients[22] exist in relation to doctors and nurses. Patients are under authority; they are in contact with the service because they are sick, and to become well again they should obey doctor's orders. 'Education' however implies the existence of learners. Learners can exist independently of teachers; they should be expected to take an active part in their own learning, and in adult education in particular their contribution to the learning process is recognised as being individual and valuable. 'Teaching patients', while not a contradiction in terms, certainly involves a reconsideration of the role of the non-professional partner.

Parents and prospective parents are in a slightly different position from the more usual patient. Staff concerned with patients in these fields are well aware that the nature of their work is different from nursing the sick. Midwifery is a separate profession from nursing, though most midwives are also qualified as nurses. Midwives have patients, but they point out that their patients are not sick. Health visitors, with their public health background and their complicated relationship with social work,[23] frequently avoid the word 'patients' and talk about 'clients', 'caseloads' or simply 'mothers'. Sociologists debate about the extent to which pregnant women behave as if they were sick, and differ about whether research findings reveal characteristics of the women concerned, or of pregnancy, or of the way in which the health services process pregnant women.[24] Clearly, pregnant women are not normal patients. Parents consulting a professional about their children are not really patients at all; it is the child who is the patient, and the parent has the job of recognising the existence of a problem,[25] reporting it to the professional, and discussing the possible management of the child. However doctors and nurses treat pregnant women, pregnancy is still in most cases a normal physiological process; however doctors and nurses treat parents of small children, the parents are still responsible for the day to day management of that child, unless the child is sick enough to be admitted to hospital.

This is patently a complicated situation, and it may be that its very complexity has resulted in the explicit teaching tradition among health service staff who deal with parents and prospective parents. For these patient groups retain considerable control over their own actions, and it is interesting that those professional groups which take most readily to educational work appear to be those whose power over patients is clearly limited.[26] If the process in question can be controlled only or mainly by the patient, the staff have a motive for undertaking education, and the patient one for receiving it. The issue of control applies not only to the process, but also to the balance of power in relationships. Successful education involves not only activity on the part of the teacher, but even more important, activity on the part of the learner. In a relationship where communication is controlled by the professional, the patient is less likely to play an active part in his own learning. The greater the perceived power of the professional group, and the more impressive the technological apparatus, the more likely the patient is to accept blindly the professional's control of the encounter and not make much effort to learn. Midwives, nurses and paramedical groups are far better placed than doctors to undertake patient education precisely because their perceived power is less than that of doctors, and they may therefore be seen as more approachable. Thus one woman commented on her community midwife: 'I felt very at ease with her, and I could ask her anything and know I would get an answer'.[27]

Asking questions is a promising first step for patients to take part in their own learning. Developments from this starting point, however, may depend on the professionals concerned encouraging patient initiative and patient participation. In maternity work, and in most work with children, it is obvious that the parents will have to take over the process eventually. In other specialities, the need for patient initiative may be less immediately apparent. However, others besides enthusiasts for patient education have an interest in patient participation and individual treatment. The nursing process, for example, represents an attempt to plan and give individualised nursing care. Care plans, it has been argued, should be developed after systematic assessment of a patient's needs, psychological and social as well as physical, and should be developed in co-operation with individual patients, not independently of them. What this may involve in practice is illustrated by Wendy Hannan's account of developing a care plan for Mr M, partially paralysed after an accident at work four years ago and admitted to hospital for 24 hours for routine investigations.

> *It . . . seemed ludicrous to me to attempt to nurse Mr M without consulting him.* He was, after four years' personal experience, in a much better position than I to know his problems and the intervention that should be taken . . . In view of this I resolved to explain to Mr M my appreciation of his long experience and ask his advice as to the best possible way of looking after him. *It was a little difficult openly to admit a lack of knowledge, but it seemed the most sensible, logical and caring thing to do.*[28] (Author's italics)

This short extract shows that some of the issues which have been discussed at length in the context of patient education also arise in nursing care. Patients have a distinctive and valuable contribution to make to their own learning and to their own care. Those who are in a position to teach them, or to care for them, may find it difficult at first to ask for this contribution to be made, but it is 'the most sensible, logical, caring thing to do'. In some situations patient education can contribute to the success of nursing care; in others nursing care may be incomplete without patient education. Other settings require other studies; this book has been concerned with only a limited number of settings, and with a particular, idiosyncratic, type of patient — parents and prospective parents.

Progress and Practicalities

This book has argued for evolution not revolution. Detailed examination of health service teaching practice shows the possibilities open to those professionals who wish to improve their teaching skills, and those parents who wish to learn. Improvements are possible without drastic upheavals in health service organisation; this can be seen both from evidence of good teaching practice in the health service, and by envisaging developments from existing practice which involve comparatively little additional expense. For such improvements to take place, however, there are certain requirements which relate to attitudes and not to money. To start with, it is necessary to accept that practice in the health service has not yet been made perfect. 'But we do all that already' is a predictable response from some members of any profession to suggestions for developments from existing traditions. It is also a difficult response for an innovator to handle, since it may be true. It may also, however, be based on a misunderstanding of what is proposed, or a failure to examine existing practice with sufficient precision and detachment to see what actually is being done, and what is not. Such examination needs to be local, and at times individual, rather than national, large scale and therefore general. It is not enough to say, when faced with yet another survey showing patient dissatisfaction with the level of information in X hospital, that 'of course it doesn't happen here'. One must ask such a protester: 'How do you know, if you haven't asked? How do you know, if you have no plans to see that it doesn't? How do you know, if you haven't checked recently?' It is hoped that readers will not dismiss the local studies in this volume as being untypical, without checking first to see precisely what is happening in their own area.

The second requirement is a willingness to identify and tackle soluble problems rather than insoluble ones. Some potential settings for health service teaching may never even approach perfection, because, for example, the demands of clinical work are too pressing to allow their possibilities for teaching to be realised — at least without, say, doubling the numbers of staff employed. Where this is the case, it is sensible to identify and act on any marginal improvements that can be made, and then look for more practical alternatives elsewhere.

The third requirement is that those who are responsible for health service teaching are clinically competent, do in fact wish to teach in such a way as to meet individual need, and are prepared to work with their patients to achieve the learning which is their common aim.

Throughout this book I have taken clinical competence for granted. My own experience of working with health service staff has led me to believe that, in general, practitioners do wish to meet patient need, and that therefore what I am suggesting is indeed evolution, not revolution; a matter of acquiring new techniques and new perspective, not new principles. Progress in patient education can thus be seen as a natural process of maturation, not a grafting of alien tissue or an invasive growth. This book has examined some of the factors which foster or retard its healthy development in practice.

Notes

1. Documented in the study of antenatal class provision discussed in Chapter 5.
2. Elizabeth R. Perkins, 'And Did You Go to Classes, Mrs Brown?', *Midwives' Chronicle and Nursing Notes* (December 1979), pp. 422-5.
3. Hilary Graham, 'Problems in Antenatal Care', paper presented at the Child Poverty Action Group Conference, 'Reaching the Consumer in the Antenatal and Child Health Services' (York, 1978).
4. Report of the Committee on Child Health Services, *Fit for the Future* (HMSO, London, 1976).
5. Elizabeth R. Perkins, 'Antenatal Care and Postnatal Nursing: Aspects of the Role of the Midwife in Health Education' in D.C. Anderson (ed.), *Health Education in Practice* (Croom Helm, London, 1979).
6. Ursula Inman, *Towards a Theory of Nursing Care* (Royal College of Nursing, London, 1975).
7. Perkins, 'Antenatal Care and Postnatal Nursing'.
8. Suggestions for methods are given in Elizabeth R. Perkins and D.C. Anderson, *Self Assessment in the NHS: Techniques for Monitoring and Research* (Nafferton Books, Driffield, 1980); Elizabeth R. Perkins, 'Monitoring Antenatal Classes: The Development of a Research Tool', *Nursing Times*, vol. 75 (13 December 1979), pp. 2163-7; J. M. Clark and L. Hockey, *Research for Nursing: A Guide for the Enquiring Nurse* (HM & M, Aylesbury, 1979), pp. 78-92.
9. J. Prince and M.E. Adams, *Minds, Mothers and Midwives: The Psychology of Childbirth* (Churchill Livingstone, Edinburgh, 1978), is a good example of the use of psychological findings to help professionals to understand patients' needs.
10. This is a matter of academic debate; see, for example, J.W. Donovan *et al.*, 'Routine Advice against Smoking in Pregnancy', *Journal of the Royal College of General Practitioners*, vol. 25 (1975), pp. 264-8; L. Baric, Christine MacArthur and M. Sherwood, 'A Study of Health Education Aspects of Smoking in Pregnancy', *International Journal of Health Education*, supplement to vol. XIX, no. 2 (April-June 1976); J.W. Donovan, 'Randomised Controlled Trial of Anti-smoking Advice in Pregnancy', *British Journal of Preventive and Social Medicine*, vol. 31 (1977), pp. 6-12.
11. For reviews of the literature, see Debra L. Roter, 'Patient Participation in the Patient-provider Interaction: The Effects of Patient Question Asking on the Quality of Interaction, Satisfaction and Compliance', *Health Education Monographs* (Winter 1977), p. 281; and Clark and Hockey, *Research for Nursing*.
12. M.L.J. Abercrombie and P.M. Terry, 'Talking to Learn: Improving Teaching and Learning in Small Groups', Research into Higher Education

Monographs (Society for Research into Higher Education, University of Surrey, 1978).

13. Sheila Hillier, 'Situational Stress and Smoking among Student Nurses – An Educational Approach', paper given at the Health Educational Council Workshop on Health Education in Nursing Practice (Eastbourne, 1979).

14. Examples of midwives' teaching which were shaming in their effect are included in Perkins, 'Antenatal Care and Postnatal Nursing'.

15. Sonya J. Hermann, *Becoming Assertive: A Guide for Nurses* (D. van Nostrand Company, New York, 1978).

16. Isabel E.P. Menzies, 'The Functioning of Social Systems as a Defence Against Anxiety', Tavistock Pamphlet no. 3 (Tavistock Institute of Human Relations, London, 1970). The point is repeated in Margot Jefferys, 'A Study of the Relationship between Situational Stress and the Smoking Habits of Nurses in Three Selected Hospitals', end of grant report to the SSRC (June 1974).

17. E. Cassee, 'Therapeutic Behaviour, Hospital Culture and Communication' in Caroline Cox and Adrianne Mead (eds.), *A Sociology of Medical Practice* (Collier-Macmillan, London, 1975), discusses the effect of relationships between hospital staff on relationships between staff and patients.

18. L. Baric, in 'Evaluation', paper given at the Tenth International Conference of Health Education (London, September 1979), argues that evaluation in health education lacks theoretical models of health behaviour, and methods of assessing the informal health education, which takes place outside the sphere of professional control. The limitations of current evaluative research are shown in A. Gatherer *et al.*, *Is Health Education Effective?* (Health Educational Council, London, 1979).

19. A further argument for health education is that which favours a raising of the general levels of health knowledge, and the setting of expectations for the behaviour of particular groups. Thus L. Baric and C. MacArthur, 'Health Norms in Pregnancy', *British Journal of Preventive and Social Medicine*, vol. 31 (1977), pp. 30-8, describe the power of norms of appropriate behaviour in pregnancy to influence women's behaviour with regard to diet, exercise, drugs and alcohol, and argue that the norm concerning smoking in pregnancy is not yet generally accepted as having coercive power. They suggest that health education should be directed, not solely at the 'at risk group', but at those who will influence their behaviour by their disapproval. This argument is related to the wish to change the attitudes of a population, rather than merely to convey information directly to change individuals' behaviour. While it is of considerable interest to those whose focus is on a large population, it has little direct relevance to the situation of health service staff faced with individual patients, or small groups of patients, who are pregnant and smoking, unless the staff also have regular access to other members of the family and can persuade them to exert pressure on the pregnant woman to stop smoking.

20. Hilary Graham, 'Smoking in Pregnancy: The Attitudes of Expectant Mothers', *Social Science and Medicine*, vol. 10 (1976), pp. 399-405.

21. Teaching adults to use the techniques of behaviour modification to help them to change their habits features in the Open University course, *Health Choices* (1980).

22. The conceptual difficulties in the word 'patient' and the available alternatives are discussed in Margaret Stacey, 'The Health Service Consumer: A Sociological Misconception', *Sociological Review Monograph*, vol. 22 (1976), p. 194.

23. June Clark, *A Family Visitor* (Royal College of Nursing, London, 1973), states: 'The health visitors were unable to describe with any precision the difference between health visiting and social work.'

24. W.R. Rosengren, 'Social Sources of Pregnancy as Illness or Normality', *Social Forces*, vol. 39 (1961), p. 260; John B. McKinley, 'The Sick Role – Illness and Pregnancy', *Social Science and Medicine*, vol. 6 (1972), p. 561; Warren M. Hern, 'The Illness Parameters of Pregnancy', *Social Science and Medicine*, vol. 9 (1975), p. 365; Ann Oakley, 'The Trap of Medicalised Motherhood', *New Society* (18 December 1975), p. 639; Ann Oakley, *Becoming a Mother* (Martin Robertson, Oxford, 1979).

25. N.J. Spencer, 'Aspects of Illness-related Decision-making by Parents of Small Children', Occasional Paper 10 (Leverhulme Health Education Project, University of Nottingham, 1978).

26. Outside the maternity and child health service, for example, physiotherapists and dietitians have established teaching traditions.

27. A comment from a mother of a six-week-old baby, describing her community midwife as the most helpful person she had met over the period of pregnancy, delivery and the return home; collected as part of the survey outlined in Perkins, 'Antenatal Care and Postnatal Nursing'.

28. 'Rediscovering the Patient', *Nursing Times Supplement* (30 November 1978), in particular Wendy Hannan, 'Introduction to Planning Care', pp. 5-7; and Pat Ashworth, G. Castledine and Jean K. McFarlane, 'The Process in Practice', pp. 3-4.

Abercrombie, M.L.J. and Terry, P.M. 'Talking to Learn: Improving Teaching and Learning in Small Groups', Research into Higher Education Monographs (Society for Research into Higher Education, University of Surrey, 1978)

Anderson D.C. 'Abstractive and Observational Methods of Educational Evaluation in a Dietetic Clinic', paper read at the 10th International Conference of Health Education (London, September, 1979)

—— (ed.) *Health Education in Practice* (Croom Helm, London, 1979)

—— 'The Practical Implementation of a Health Education Programme' in Anderson (ed.) *Health Education in Practice*

—— 'Talking with Patients about their Diet' in Anderson (ed.) *Health Education in Practice*

—— *Evaluation by Classroom Experience* (Nafferton Books, Driffield, 1979)

—— 'Systematic and Modest Schemes for Health Education in Schools' in Anderson (ed.) *The Ignorance of Social Intervention* (Croom Helm, London, 1980)

Anderson, D.C., Perkins, E.R. and Spencer, N.J. 'Who Knows Best in Health Education?', Occasional Paper 19 (Leverhulme Health Education Project, University of Nottingham, 1979)

Anderson, J.A.D. and Gatherer, A. 'Hygiene of Infant Feeding Utensils: Practice and Standards in the Home', *British Medical Journal*, vol. 2 (1970), pp. 20-3

Ashworth, P., Castledine, G. and McFarlane, J.K. 'The Process in Practice' in 'Rediscovering the Patient', *Nursing Times Supplement* (30 November 1978), pp. 3-4

Baric, L. 'Evaluation', paper read at the 10th International Conference of Health Education (London, September 1979)

Baric , L. and MacArthur, C. 'Health Norms in Pregnancy', *British Journal of Preventive and Social Medicine*, vol. 31 (1977), pp. 30-8

Baric, L., MacArthur, C. and Sherwood, M. 'A Study of Health Education Aspects of Smoking in Pregnancy', *International Journal of Health Education*, supplement to vol. XIX, no. 2 (April-June 1976)

Becker, H.S. *Sociological Work: Method and Substance* (Allen Lane, London, 1971)

Becker, H.S., Everett, B., Hughes, G. and Strauss, A.L. *Boys in White: Student Culture in Medical School* (Chicago University Press,

Chicago, 1961)

Beels, C. *The Childbirth Book* (Turnstone Books, London, 1978)

Benson, H. with Klipper, M.Z. *The Relaxation Response* (Collins, London, 1976)

Bloor, M. 'Professional Autonomy and Client Exclusion: A Study in ENT Clinics' in Wadsworth and Robinson (eds.) *Studies in Everyday Medical Life*

Bradshaw, J.S. 'A Taxonomy of Social Need' in McLachlan (ed.) *Problems and Progress in Medical Care: Essays on Current Research*, 7th series

Brammer, A.E. 'Report of an Enquiry into Organised Classes for Pregnant Women and their Partners provided by the Maternity Services in England in 1975' (unpublished report, Royal College of Midwives, London, 1977)

Breese, A.C. 'Antenatal Classes and Preparation for Pregnancy, Birth and Motherhood' (unpublished MMedSci dissertation, University of Nottingham, 1976)

Brown, G.W. 'Social Causes of Disease' in Tuckett (ed.) *An Introduction to Medical Sociology*

Byrne, P. and Long, B. *Doctors Talking to Patients* (HMSO, London, 1976)

Cartwright, A. *Human Relations and Hospital Care* (Routledge & Kegan Paul, London, 1964)

Cassee, E. 'Therapeutic Behaviour, Hospital Culture and Communication' in Cox and Mead (eds.) *A Sociology of Medical Practice*

Chamberlain, G. 'Antenatal Education', *Midwife, Health Visitor and Community Nurse*, vol. 11 (September 1975), p. 289

Chamberlain, G. and Chave, S. 'Antenatal Education', *Community Health (Bristol)*, vol. 9 (1977), p. 11

Chard, T. and Richards, M. (eds.) *Benefits and Hazards of the New Obstetrics: Clinics in Developmental Medicine*, no. 64 (Heinemann, in association with Spastics International Medical Publications, London, 1977)

Chertok, L. *Motherhood and Personality, Psychosomatic Aspects of Childbirth*, English edition (Tavistock, London, 1969)

Cicourel, A.V. *Method and Measurement in Sociology* (Free Press, New York, 1964)

Clark, J. *A Family Visitor* (Royal College of Nursing, London, 1973)

Clark, J.M. and Hockey, L. *Research for Nursing: A Guide for the Enquiring Nurse* (HM & M, Aylesbury, 1979)

Comaroff, J. 'Conflicting Paradigms of Pregnancy: Managing Ambi-

guity in Antenatal Encounters' in Davies and Horobin (eds.)
Medical Encounters: The Experience of Illness and Treatment
Committee on Child Health Services *Fit for the Future* (HMSO,
London, 1976)
Cox, C. and Mead, A. (eds.) *A Sociology of Medical Practice* (Collier-
Macmillan, London, 1975)
Craven, R.O., Crouch, M. and Goosey, R.A. 'Guidelines for Teachers of
Parentcraft and Relaxation', *Midwives' Chronicle and Nursing Notes*
(January-August 1975)
Davies, A. and Horobin, G. (eds.) *Medical Encounters: The Experience
of Illness and Treatment* (Croom Helm, London, 1977)
Davies, D.P. 'Osmolality Homeostasis and Renal Function in Infancy',
Postgraduate Medical Journal, vol. 51, supplement 3 (1975), pp. 25-30
Deutsch, H. *The Psychology of Women: A Psychoanalytic Interpretation,
Motherhood*, vol. 2 (Research Books, London, 1947)
Department of Health and Social Security *Present Day Practice in Infant
Feeding*, Report on Health and Social Subjects, no. 9 (HMSO,
London, 1974)
—— *The Family and Society: Dimensions of Parenthood* (HMSO, London,
1974)
Dick Read, G. *Natural Childbirth* (Heinemann, London, 1933)
Donovan, J.W. 'Randomised Controlled Trial of Anti-smoking Advice in
Pregnancy', *British Journal of Preventive and Social Medicine*, vol. 31
(1977), pp. 6-12
Donovan, J.W., *et al.* 'Routine Advice against Smoking in Pregnancy',
Journal of the Royal College of General Practitioners, vol. 25 (1975),
pp. 264-8
Driscoll, K.O., Strange, J.M. and Minogue, M. 'Active Management of
Labour', *British Medical Journal*, vol. 3 (1977), pp. 135-7
Emmett Holt, L. *Care and Feeding of Infants* (D. Appleton & Co.,
New York and London, 1896)
Farnes, N. (ed.) *Community Education with the Open University*,
provisional edition (Open University, Milton Keynes, May 1979)
Fenwick, P. and Fenwick, C. *The Baby Book for Fathers* (Angus &
Robertson, Brighton, 1978)
Gatherer, A., *et al. Is Health Education Effective?* (Health Education
Council, London, 1979)
Gillett, J.R. 'Helping Those Who Have Not Been to Preparation for
Childbirth Classes', *Midwives' Chronicle and Nursing Notes*,
(February 1977), pp. 32-3
Goody, E.M. 'Parental Roles in Anthropological Perspective' in

Department of Health and Social Security, *The Family and Society: Dimensions of Parenthood*

Graham, H. 'Smoking in Pregnancy: The Attitudes of Expectant Mothers', *Social Science and Medicine*, vol. 10 (1976), pp. 399-405
—— 'Problems in Antenatal Care', paper presented at the Child Poverty Action Group Conference, 'Reaching the Consumer in the Antenatal and Child Health Services' (York, 1978)
—— *The First Months of Motherhood* (University of York, 1979)

Haire, D. 'The Cultural Warping of Childbirth', *ICEA News Special Issue* (Washington, 1972)

Hannan, W. 'Introduction to Planning Care' in 'Rediscovering the Patient', *Nursing Times Supplement* (30 November 1978), pp. 5-7

Hassid, P. *Textbook for Childbirth Educators* (Harper & Row, Hagerstown, Maryland, 1978)

Henry, S. 'The Dangers of Self-help Groups', *New Society* (22 June 1978), p. 654.

Hermann, S.J. *Becoming Assertive: A Guide for Nurses* (D. van Nostrand Company, New York, 1978)

Hern, W.M. 'The Illness Parameters of Pregnancy', *Social Science and Medicine*, vol. 9 (1975), p. 365

Hibbard, B.M., *et al.* 'The Effectiveness of Antenatal Education', *Health Education Journal*, vol. 38, no. 2 (1979), pp. 39-46

Hillier, S. 'Situational Stress and Smoking among Student Nurses – An Educational Approach', paper given at the Health Education Council Workshop on Health Education in Nursing Practice (Eastbourne, 1979)

Houghton, H. 'Problems of Hospital Communication' in McLachlan (ed.) *Problems and Progress in Medical Care: Essays on Current Research*, 3rd series

Hutchinson-Smith, B. 'The Relationship between the Weight of an Infant and Lower Respiratory Infection', *Medical Officer*, vol. 123 (1970), pp. 257-62

Illingworth, R.S. and Illingworth, C. *Babies and Young Children*, 6th edn (Churchill Livingstone, Edinburgh, 1978)

Inman, U. *Towards a Theory of Nursing Care* (Royal College of Nursing, London, 1975)

Jefferys, M. 'A Study of the Relationship between Situational Stress and the Smoking Habits of Nurses in Three Selected Hospitals', end of grant report to the SSRC (June 1974)

Kitzinger, S. *Education and Counselling for Childbirth* (Baillière Tindall, London, 1977)

—— *The Good Birth Guide* (Fontana, Glasgow, 1979)

Kitzinger, S. and Davis, J. (eds.) *The Place of Birth* (Oxford University Press, Oxford, 1978)

Korsch, B.M., Gozzi, E.M. and Francis, V. 'Gaps in Doctor-patient Communication', *Pediatrics*, vol. 42, no. 5 (November 1968), pp. 855-71

Lawton, J.W. and Shortridge, K.F. 'Protective Factors in Human Breast Milk and Colostrum', *Lancet*, vol. 1 (January 1977), p. 253

Leach, P. *Babyhood* (Pelican Books, London, 1974)

—— *Baby and Child* (Michael Joseph, London, 1977)

Lennane, J. and Lennane, J. *Hard Labour* (Gollancz, London, 1974)

MacLean, G.D. 'An Appraisal of the Concepts of Infant Feeding and their Application in Practice', *Journal of Advanced Nursing*, vol. 2 (1977), pp. 111-26

Mandelstam, D.A. 'The Value of Antenatal Preparation — A Statistical Survey', *Midwife and Health Visitor*, vol. 7 (June 1971), p. 217

Martin, J. *Infant Feeding 1975: Attitudes and Practice in England and Wales* (HMSO, London, 1978)

McKean, K.S., Baum, J.D. and Sloper, K.D. 'Factors Influencing Breast Feeding', *Archives of Disease in Childhood*, vol. 50, no. 3 (March 1975), pp. 165-70

McKinley, J.B. 'The Sick Role — Illness and Pregnancy', *Social Science and Medicine*, vol. 6 (1972), p. 561

McLachlan, G. (ed.) *Problems and Progress in Medical Care: Essays on Current Research*, 3rd series (Oxford University Press, London, 1968)

—— *Problems and Progress in Medical Care: Essays on Current Research*, 7th series (Oxford University Press, London, 1972)

Menzies, I.E.P. 'The Functioning of Social Systems and a Defence against Anxiety', Tavistock Pamphlet no. 3 (Tavistock Institute of Human Relations, London, 1970)

Ministry of Health, Report of a Working Party on the Field of Work, Training and Recruitment of Health Visitors 'An Enquiry into Health Visiting' (London, 1950)

Newson, J. and Newson, E. *Patterns of Infant Care in an Urban Community* (Allen & Unwin, London, 1963)

—— *Four Years Old in an Urban Community* (Allen & Unwin, London, 1968)

—— *Seven Years Old in the Home Environment* (Allen & Unwin, London, 1976)

Oakley, A 'The Baby Blues', *New Society* (5 April 1979), p. 11

—— 'The Trap of Medicalised Motherhood', *New Society* (18 December 1979), p. 639

—— *Becoming a Mother* (Martin Robertson, Oxford, 1979)

Open University *The First Years of Life* (Milton Keynes, 1977)

—— *The Preschool Child* (Milton Keynes, 1977)

—— *Research Methods in Education and the Social Sciences* (Milton Keynes, 1978)

—— *Health Choices* (Milton Keynes, 1980)

Owen, B. and Portress, M. 'Prospective Investigation into Cot Deaths', *Health Visitor*, vol. 48 (October 1975), p. 379

Perkins, E.R. (ed.) 'Survey of New Mothers in Sutton-in-Ashfield', mimeo (Leverhulme Health Education Project, University of Nottingham, 1976)

—— 'Having a Baby: An Educational Experience?', Occasional Paper 6 (Leverhulme Health Education Project, University of Nottingham, 1978)

—— 'Antenatal Classes in Nottinghamshire: The Pattern of Official Provision', Occasional Paper 9 (Leverhulme Health Education Project, University of Nottingham, 1978)

—— 'Antenatal Care and Postnatal Nursing: Aspects of the Role of the Midwife in Health Education' in Anderson (ed.) *Health Education in Practice*

—— 'Attendance at Antenatal Classes: A District Study', Occasional Paper 13 (Leverhulme Health Education Project, University of Nottingham, 1979)

—— 'Defining the Need: An Analysis of Varying Teaching Goals in Antenatal Classes', *International Journal of Nursing Studies*, vol. 16 (1979), pp. 275-82

—— 'Parentcraft: A Comparative Study of Teaching Method', Occasional Paper 16 (Leverhulme Health Education Project, University of Nottingham, 1979)

—— 'Monitoring Antenatal Classes: The Development of a Research Tool', *Nursing Times*, vol. 75 (13 December 1979), pp. 2163-7

—— 'And Did You Go to Classes, Mrs Brown?', *Midwives' Chronicle and Nursing Notes* (December 1979), pp. 422-5

—— 'The Pattern of Women's Attendance at Antenatal Classes: Is This Good Enough?', *Health Education Journal* (1980, in press)

Perkins, E.R. and Anderson, D.C. *Self Assessment in the NHS: Techniques for Monitoring and Research* (Nafferton Books, Driffield, 1980)

Phillips, D. *Knowledge from What?* (Rand McNally, Chicago, 1971)

Poskitt, E.M.E. and Cole, T.J. 'Nature, Nurture and Childhood Over-
    weight', *British Medical Journal*, vol. 1 (1978), pp. 603-5
Prince, J. and Adams, M.E. *Minds, Mothers and Midwives: The
    Psychology of Childbirth* (Churchill Livingstone, Edinburgh, 1978)
Rogers, E. and Shoemaker, F.F. *The Communication of Innovations*
    (Free Press, New York, 1971)
Roghmann, K.J. and Haggerty, R.J. 'Daily Stress, Illness and Use of
    Health Services in Young Families', *Paediatric Research*, vol. 7
    (1973), pp. 520-6
Rosen, M. 'Pain and its Relief' in Chard and Richards (eds.) *Benefits
    and Hazards of the New Obstetrics: Clinics in Developmental
    Medicine*, no. 64
Rosengren, W.R. 'Social Sources of Pregnancy as Illness or Normality',
    Social Forces, vol. 39 (1961), p. 260
Roter, D.L. 'Patient Participation in the Patient-provider Interaction:
    The Effects of Patient Question Asking on the Quality of Inter-
    action, Satisfaction and Compliance', *Health Education Monographs*
    (Winter, 1977), p. 281
Royal College of General Practitioners 'The Future General Practitioner:
    Learning and Teaching' (RCGP, London, 1972)
—— 'The Education of Patients and Public by General Practitioners in
    the Seventies' (unpublished study group report, 1976)
Schatzman, L. and Strauss, A.L. *Field Research: Strategies for a
    Natural Sociology* (Prentice Hall, Englewood Cliffs, New Jersey,
    1973)
Schutz, A. 'On Phenomenology and Social Relations' in Wagner (ed.)
    Selected Writings
Sharrock, W.W. 'Portraying the Professional Relationship' in Anderson
    (ed.) *Health Education in Practice*
Shaw, N.S. *Forced Labour: Maternity Care in the United States*
    (Pergamon, Oxford, 1974)
Shields, D. 'Nursing Care in Labour and Patient Satisfaction: A
    Descriptive Study', *Journal of Advanced Nursing*, vol. 3 (1978),
    pp. 535-50
Spencer, N.J. 'Aspects of Illness-related Decision-making by Parents of
    Small Children', Occasional Paper 10 (Leverhulme Health Education
    Project, University of Nottingham, 1978)
—— 'The Identification and Management of Illness by Parents of
    Young Children' (unpublished MPhil thesis, University of Nottingham,
    1980)
Spencer, N.J. and Perkins, E.R. *Evaluating Communication with Patients:*

Self Assessment Techniques for Doctors (Nafferton Books, Driffield, 1980)

Spock, B. *Baby and Child Care* (Bodley Head, London, 1958)

Stacey, M. 'The Health Service Consumer: A Sociological Misconception', *Sociological Review Monograph*, vol. 22 (1976), p. 194

Stacey, M. with Homans, H. 'The Sociology of Health and Illness: Its Present State, Future Prospects and Potential for Health Research', *Sociology*, vol. 12 (1978), p. 281

Sudnow, D. *Passing On: The Social Organisation of Dying* (Prentice Hall, Englewood Cliffs, New Jersey, 1967)

Taitz, L.S. and Byers, H.D. 'High Coloria/osmolen Feeding and Hypertonic Dehydration', *Archives of Disease in Childhood*, vol. 47 (1972), p. 257

Tuckett, D. (ed.) *An Introduction to Medical Sociology* (Tavistock, London, 1967)

Wadsworth, M. 'Studies in Doctor-patient Communication' in Wadsworth and Robinson (eds.) *Studies in Everyday Medical Life*

Wadsworth, M. and Robinson, D. (eds.) *Studies in Everyday Medical Life* (Martin Robertson, London, 1976)

Wagner, H.R. (ed.) *Selected Writings* (Chicago Press, Chicago, 1971)

Weider, D.L. *Language and Social Reality* (Mouton, The Hague, 1974)

Williams, M. and Booth, D. *Antenatal Education: Guidelines for Teachers* (Churchill Livingstone, Edinburgh, 1974)

INDEX

For Product Safety Concerns and Information please contact our EU
representative GPSR@taylorandfrancis.com
Taylor & Francis Verlag GmbH, Kaufingerstraße 24, 80331 München, Germany

www.ingramcontent.com/pod-product-compliance
Lightning Source LLC
Chambersburg PA
CBHW050714280326
41926CB00088B/3027